THE
RAPID
WAIST
REDUCTION
DIET

DON COLBERT, MD

SILOAM

Most Charisma House Book Group products are available at special quantity discounts for bulk purchase for sales promotions, premiums, fund-raising, and educational needs. For details, write Charisma House Book Group, 600 Rinehart Road, Lake Mary, Florida 32746, or telephone (407) 333-0600.

The Rapid Waist Reduction Diet
   by Don Colbert, MD
Published by Siloam
Charisma Media/Charisma House Book Group
600 Rinehart Road, Lake Mary, Florida 32746
www.charismahouse.com

Cover design by Justin Evans
Design Director: Bill Johnson

Visit the author's website at www.drcolbert.com.

Library of Congress Cataloging-in-Publication Data:
An application to register this book for cataloging has been submitted to the Library of Congress.
International Standard Book Number: 978-1-62136-044-5
E-book ISBN: 978-1-62136-045-2

Contents

Introduction

IT'S ALL ABOUT
"WAIST MANAGEMENT"

G OD'S DESIRE IS for you to feel better and to live longer—and He will help you reach that goal! By picking up this book you have taken a major step toward renewed energy and health. This book can help you restore your health and get rid of the toxic belly fat that leads to disease and ill health.

Losing weight may be the greatest physical challenge of your life. But with faith in God, good nutrition, and cutting-edge natural remedies, reducing your waistline can represent a great victory in your life! God revealed His divine will for each of us through the apostle John, who wrote, "Beloved, I pray that you may prosper in all things and be in health, just as your soul prospers" (3 John 2).

It's no secret that America has been experiencing a rise in obesity for several years now. What's alarming is that we've reached epidemic proportions: two-thirds of American adults are overweight or obese, and 30 percent of children age eleven or younger are overweight.[1] This ought to alarm everyone, particularly everyone who professes Jesus as Savior and Lord. Surely we are missing

God's best. Why? The conventional answer is that many physicians are looking for the next new-and-improved medication. I suggest that is not a solution. We need to get to the *root* of the problem, which is our diet, lifestyle, and waistline. Without addressing this reality, the alarming toll from obesity will only get worse.

Fast food, junk food, convenience foods, sodas, sweetened coffee drinks, sugar-laden juices, smoothies, "supersize" portions, and skipping meals all contribute to the problem. The standard American diet is full of empty carbohydrates, sugars, fats, excessive proteins, and calories, and it is low in nutrient content. This diet literally causes us to lose nutrients such as chromium, which is crucial in regulating glucose levels in our blood.

Combined with our poor diet is a lack of physical activity. Too many children no longer play sports and participate in outdoor activities. Instead they get entranced by video games, smartphones, text messages, social networking, online media, TV, and movies. Combined with their favorite fast food, reducing exercise to a flick of the finger on a remote control spells ever-increasing weight gain.

Also, the excessive stress that most adults and many children labor under increases cortisol levels. As a result, many are developing toxic belly fat, thereby increasing their risk for incurring diabetes and other diseases. Long-term stress eventually depletes stress hormones as well as neurotransmitters. This often helps unleash ravenous appetites, plus addictions to sugar and carbohydrates. It's like a nightmarish vortex, each bad habit working to ensnare sufferers in a downward spiral to poor health and disease.

YOUR WEIGHT IS YOUR CHOICE

Galatians 6:7–8 says, "Do not be deceived, God is not mocked; for whatever a man sows, that he will also reap. For he who sows to his flesh will of the flesh reap corruption, but he who sows to the Spirit will of the Spirit reap everlasting life." Most Americans are unknowingly sowing seeds for a harvest of obesity, diabetes, and a host of other diseases by their choices of food and lifestyle habits.

I often say that obesity-related diseases are "choice" diseases. In other words, you *catch* a cold or the flu, but because of wrong choices you *develop* obesity, type 2 diabetes, and other diseases.

Hosea 4:6 says, "My people are destroyed for lack of knowledge." My previous books *The Seven Pillars of Health* and *Dr. Colbert's "I Can Do This" Diet* provide a foundation for changing dietary patterns, improving lifestyle habits, and losing weight—especially toxic belly fat. I encourage you to read *The Seven Pillars of Health.* The principles it contains are a foundation for healthy living that will affect all areas of your life. It sets the stage for everything you will ever read in any other book I've published, including this one.

In this book, *The Rapid Waist Reduction Diet*, you will learn about natural ways to shrink your waist size and lose belly fat through diet, supplements, and exercise. There is hope! Your body is fearfully and wonderfully made. God can heal your body without difficulty. I have known people who were healed by God's miracle-working power. I have witnessed others whose lives have dramatically improved through healthy lifestyle choices and natural treatments. Realize that God generally won't do what you can do yourself. After all, only you can choose to eat healthy foods, exercise, lose weight, and take supplements.

Since being introduced in *Reversing Diabetes*, the Rapid Waist Reduction Diet has now been refined, updated, and expanded for everyone who wants to live a healthier, longer life by taking control of their weight. In *The Rapid Waist Reduction Diet* I offer medical information and practical insights on ways to reduce your waistline, control your weight, and rid yourself of the toxic belly fat that leads to so many diseases.

There is much you can do to change the course of your health. Now is the time to run to the battle with fresh confidence, renewed determination, and the wonderful knowledge that God is real, alive, and more powerful than any sickness or disease. It is my prayer that my suggestions and guidelines will help improve your health, nutritional habits, and fitness practices. This combination will bring wholeness to your life. I pray that they will deepen your fellowship with God and strengthen your ability to worship and serve Him.

—Don Colbert, MD

Chapter 1

THE OBESITY
EPIDEMIC

WHEN NEW YORK filmmaker Morgan Spurlock set out to draw a line between the rise of obesity in America and fast-food giant McDonald's, he never dreamed that his *Super Size Me* documentary would be nominated for an Academy Award, earn more than $20 million worldwide on a $65,000 production budget, and turn the film's title into a watchword for health activists around the globe. In short, he became McDonald's worst nightmare, one accentuated by the release of his ensuing memoir, *Don't Eat This Book.*

Spurlock's unexpected entry into international consciousness originated with a personal experiment, using himself as the guinea pig. For one month he ate nothing but McDonald's food for all three meals, in the process sampling every item on the Golden Arches' menu. Whenever cashiers asked if he wanted his meal supersized, he accepted.

When I first heard of his hypothesis, I found it a bit exaggerated. That is, until I realized that his experiment represented untold millions who get the majority of their daily sustenance from fast food. Spurlock turned himself into a physical representation of these silent masses, consuming an average of 5,000 calories a day. As a result, he gained almost 25 pounds, increased his body mass index by 13 percent, raised his cholesterol to 230, and accumulated fat in his liver. He turned his experiment into a statement heard around the world.[1]

Years later I sometimes wonder if many Americans were paying attention. After reports in recent years of a stabilization in obesity rates, a report released by the Centers for Disease Control and Prevention (CDC) in the summer of 2011 showed they had inched up 1.1 percent between 2007 and 2009, leaving them at staggering levels of 33.8 percent.[2] The proportion of obese Americans is at astounding levels, about one-third or 33.8 percent.[3] Obesity currently kills an estimated four hundred thousand Americans a year and is the second-leading cause of preventable deaths in this nation.[4] The number one avoidable killer? Cigarette smoking (and a recent report shows it dropped 40 percent between 1965 and 2007).[5] That means losing weight ranks up there with quitting smoking as the most crucial lifestyle change you could ever make. Because of the lowered smoking trend, I predict that obesity will soon pass smoking as the number one avoidable killer of Americans.

Unfortunately many doctors, nutritionists, and dietitians seem to either miss this fact or conveniently ignore it. They love to offer topical "Band-Aids" that alleviate patients' symptoms yet fail to tackle the root issues or consider the long-term ramifications of neglecting their patients' weight. A CDC report in 2007 found that about a third of obese adults had never been told by a doctor or health care provider that they were obese.[6] This is unbelievable, because obesity is also a key link to other serious, life-threatening issues such as diabetes and heart disease.

Such alarming information speaks for itself. Indeed, it is screaming while far too many practitioners turn the other way. With our nation facing the biggest health care crisis in its history, each of us must realize that the answer won't come from doctors, clinics, or the US government. Instead, each person must take responsibility for his or her health. Because obesity and belly fat are at the root of so many health conditions, it makes sense to start by reducing to a healthy weight and a healthy waistline.

DEFINING THE PROBLEM

Before I delve into what has so many people visiting the plus-size department and developing disease along the way, I need to clarify the terms *overweight* and *obese*. Many people have a general sense as to how these words are different, yet in recent years the delineation has become clearer. Various health organizations, including the CDC and the National Institutes of Health (NIH), now officially define them using the body mass index (BMI), which evaluates a person's weight relative to height. Most of these organizations define an overweight adult as having a BMI between 25 and 29.9, while an obese adult is anyone with a BMI of 30 or higher.[7]

Only a small portion of individuals who are overweight or obese according to their BMI have a normal or low body fat percentage. For example, professional athletes often have a high-muscle, low-body-fat makeup that causes them to weigh more than the average person, yet they are not truly obese (excluding some football linemen and sumo wrestlers). However, most people who come to me seeking help are not just overweight but technically obese—meaning males with body fat greater than 25 percent and females over 33 percent.[8] Throughout this book when I discuss having a high BMI, I will be referring to obese people, not those few muscular types with a high BMI but normal or low body fat.

Calories Cost

Researchers have discovered that for every extra 100 calories a person eats each day, the additional expenses—such as health care for future health problems caused by being overweight—range from forty-eight cents to two dollars. Each time you supersize your meal for "only" thirty-five cents more, it can actually end up costing you between eighty-two cents and six dollars and sixty-four cents in health care bills.

When everything is considered, obesity comes with a fat price tag (pun intended), with people considered obese paying $1,429 more (42 percent) in health care costs than normal weight individuals. Expenses for each obese senior run Medicare $1,723 more than for normal weight beneficiaries, and private insurers $1,140 more.[9]

And, as shocking as all this sounds, no dollar amount can do justice to the real damage being done. Being overweight or obese increases your risk of developing thirty-five major diseases, particularly type 2 diabetes, heart disease, stroke, arthritis, hypertension, Alzheimer's disease, infertility, erectile dysfunction, and gallbladder disease—plus more than a dozen forms of cancer. If you are an obese woman, you have a significantly higher risk of postmenopausal breast cancer—one and a half times more than a woman with an average healthy weight.[10] You also increase your chances of developing uterine cancer because of your weight.[11] For pregnant mothers, the risk of delivering a baby with a serious birth defect is doubled if you are overweight and quadrupled if you are obese.[12]

Besides obesity's physical implications, it carries a social and psychological impact. Obese individuals generally contend with more rejection and prejudice. Often they are overlooked for promotions or not even hired because of physical appearance. Most obese people struggle daily with issues of self-worth and self-image. They feel unattractive and unappreciated and are at an increased risk of depression. Many of us have watched the humiliation an obese person experiences trying to squeeze into an airplane, stadium, or automobile seat that is too small. Maybe you have been that person. If so, you know how obesity can affect the way others treat you and how you treat yourself.

GLOBESITY IS THE CULPRIT

Tragically millions of others outside the United States struggle with the same issues. The World Health Organization calls obesity a worldwide epidemic. Obesity and its expanding list of health consequences are overtaking infection and malnutrition as the main cause of death and disability in many third-world nations. This "globesity," as Morgan Spurlock aptly points out in his documentary, has a major cause: the spread of fast food.

In his award-winning *Fast Food Nation* author Eric Schlosser chronicled how Americans spent about $6 billion on fast food in 1970, but by the turn of the century shelled out more than $110 billion. Because corporate America is a global trendsetter, other countries have followed suit. Between 1984 and 1993 the number of fast-food restaurants in Great Britain doubled. So did adults' obesity rate. Fast-forward fifteen years, and the British were eating more fast food than any other nation in Western Europe.

Meanwhile the proportion of overweight teens in China has roughly tripled in the past decade. In Japan the obesity rate among children doubled during the 1980s, which correlated with a 200 percent increase in fast-food sales. This generation of Japanese has gone on to become the first in that traditionally slender Asian nation's history—thanks to its past proclivity for vegetables, rice, and fish—to be known for its bulging waistlines. By the year 2000 approximately one-third of all Japanese men in their thirties were overweight.[13] By adopting our fast-food habits, the entire world is beginning to look more like Americans. I fear that its obesity rates will soon follow.

The Link to Illnesses

- More than 90 percent of people who are newly diagnosed with type 2 diabetes are overweight or obese.[14]

- Obesity increases your risk of developing the following cancers: esophageal, thyroid, colon, kidney, prostate, endometrial, gallbladder, rectal, breast, pancreatic, leukemia, multiple myeloma, malignant melanoma, and non-Hodgkin's lymphoma.[15]

- Being overweight increases your risk of having GERD (acid reflux) symptoms by 50 percent; being obese doubles your chances.[16]

- Excess weight is also commonly known to cause sleep apnea and hypertension (high blood pressure). In fact, 75 percent of all cases of hypertension in the United States is attributed to obesity.[17]

IN THE GENES OR IN THE WATER?

Every obese person has a story behind his or her excessive weight gain. Growing up, I often heard people say things like "she was born fat" or "he takes after his daddy."

There's some truth in both comments. When it comes to obesity, genetics count.

In 1988 the *New England Journal of Medicine* published a Danish study that observed 540 people adopted during infancy. The research found that adopted individuals had a much greater tendency to end up in the weight class of their biological parents rather than their adoptive parents.[18] Separate studies of twins raised apart also show that genetics has a strong influence on weight gain and becoming overweight.[19] Such studies reveal there is a significant genetic predisposition to gaining weight.

However, they still don't fully explain the epidemic of obesity seen in the United States the past thirty years.

Although an individual may have a genetic predisposition to become obese, environment also plays a major role. I like the way author, speaker, and noted women's physician Pamela Peeke puts it: "Genetics may load the gun, but environment pulls the trigger."[20] Many patients I see come into my office thinking that since they have inherited their "fat genes," there is nothing they can do. Yet, after a little investigation, I usually find that they have inherited their parents' propensity for bad food choices, large portion sizes, and poor eating habits.

If you have been overweight since childhood, you probably have an increased number of fat cells. This means you will have a tendency to gain weight if you choose the wrong types of foods and large portions and fail to exercise. However, you should also realize that most people can override a genetic predisposition for obesity by making correct dietary and lifestyle choices. A parent's diabetes does not automatically condemn a child to the same disease, no matter how many people remark, "The apple doesn't fall far from the tree."

Unfortunately many of us forget that to make these healthy choices, we need to place ourselves in a healthy environment. That is becoming more difficult than ever as families yield to hectic routines that feature grabbing breakfast on the way out the door, fast-food lunches, dining out for dinner, and sometimes skipping meals. Years of such habits are catching up to us. Starting at age twenty-five, the average American adult gains 1 to 3 pounds a year. That means a twenty-five-year-old, 120-pound female can expect to weigh anywhere between 150 and 210 pounds by the time she is fifty-five.

Is there any wonder we have an epidemic of heart disease, type 2 diabetes, hypertension, high cholesterol, arthritis, cancer, and other degenerative diseases? We have to put the brakes on this obesity epidemic—and a lifestyle approach to eating is the answer!

EATING WITH THE HEAD, NOT THE HEART

The fact that obesity can stem from heredity, environment, and culture can feel discouraging, even overwhelming. How can one hope to overcome such powerful forces and lose belly fat in the process? As tough as it may seem, there is cause for hope. I want to end this chapter on a positive note by reminding you of a simple truth. In fact, it is one of the primary reasons for this book.

Ensalada

Just because a taco salad features the word *salad* doesn't mean it's healthy. With the massive fried tortilla shell, beef, cheese, sour cream, and additional items (plus the nutritionally useless iceberg lettuce), most taco salads add up to about 900 calories and 55 grams of fat.

It may sound impossible, but with education, practice, and discipline, your cultural tastes and dietary practices can gradually change. You can learn to choose similar foods that have not been highly processed and lower-fat alternatives. It is possible to discover—or rediscover—portion control and healthy cooking methods. What about fried chicken, mashed potatoes and gravy, and chocolate cake? You can learn to enjoy the same foods, but with just a fraction of the fat, sugar, and calories.

In an effort to help my patients I've researched many diets and eating programs over the years. As a result I've come to learn that there are two key culprits in the typical American diet that need to be addressed if you're going to lose belly fat and live a healthier life: inflammation and wheat. In the next two chapters I will discuss each of these culprits and explain why they are so detrimental to your health.

Chapter 2

CULPRIT #1:
INFLAMMATION

A FTER THE PAST decade the American Southwest could be renamed the Burning Region. Of more than two dozen major wildfires in North America since 2002, nearly 60 percent have occurred in such states as California, Nevada, New Mexico, and Arizona.

It started with the largest fire in Sequoia National Forest history in California 2002. Other blazes in the Southwest followed that killed people, burned millions of acres, destroyed thousands of homes, and caused billions of dollars worth of damage. When the largest fire in Arizona's history struck in the summer of 2011, it destroyed more than 700 square miles of land and spread into New Mexico.[1]

Every fall it seems some state in this region is bracing for another string of wildfires, hoping the winds won't blow too hard and cause the fires to spread. I remember flying over California in the autumn of 2007. I looked out my window and saw separate fires smoldering almost everywhere. It is a moment I would describe as a Salvador Dali painting come to life.

This same surreal picture describes the blazes that are

rampantly burning inside many Americans. However, unlike in the case of the Southwestern fires that held the nation's attention for weeks on end, most of us are completely unaware of what is aflame. Sadly this fire— systemic inflammation—continues to wreak havoc on millions of people, leading many toward further obesity.

What does inflammation have to do with weight gain? I want to explain their close association and examine various dietary ways that can help you curtail this inflammation.

CHRONIC INFLAMMATION AND DISEASE

Inflammation is an important component of the immune system. It is essential for the healing process since it is a programmed response, necessary for fighting infections and repairing damaged tissues. For example, when you sprain your ankle or develop tonsillitis, your white blood cells release chemicals into affected tissues. That prompts an increase in blood flow to the area, which causes redness, warmth, and pain. That is the reason your ankle or tonsils swell, become sore, and turn red. It's also why those areas heal faster. Without this response, wounds and infections would never heal. Eventually that would put your entire body at risk.

However, problems arise when this inflammatory reaction becomes systemic and goes unchecked for months or years. When this happens, the same chemicals used for healing can cause weight gain and eventually trigger a host of deadly diseases.

Localized inflammation is easy to spot and feel. Its signs include swelling, redness, warmth, and pain.

When the body triggers this healing response, you feel the pain of a strained muscle, a sprain, tendinitis, or bursitis. However, since systemic inflammation does not normally provide these symptoms, it goes unrecognized. Worse, when it is finally diagnosed, doctors and patients often dismiss it as a mere sign of aging or obesity. Unfortunately this oversight often leads to further weight gain and disease.

While chronic inflammation is a symptom of virtually every disease, it also aggravates the disease. Unremitting inflammation brings exposure to inflammatory cytokines, which are destructive, cell-signaling chemicals that contribute to most degenerative diseases. Among them are atherosclerosis, heart disease, cancer, arthritis, metabolic syndrome, Alzheimer's disease, allergies, asthma, ulcerative colitis, Crohn's disease, hepatitis, celiac disease, obesity, and diabetes.

You'll notice that almost all of these diseases are linked to obesity. Essentially, as Americans get fatter, chronic systemic inflammation increases and leads to many of these diseases. It also causes our bodies to age rapidly, including developing wrinkles.

FAT FEEDS INFLAMMATION

The obesity and inflammation connection is cyclical in nature: obesity causes increased inflammation, and increased inflammation causes more weight gain. This is partially due to fat cells manufacturing various types of inflammatory mediators, including interleukin-6, tumor necrosis factor-alpha, and plasminogen activator inhibitor-1. These all increase inflammation and are associated with atherosclerosis, or hardening of the arteries. Fat cells also produce the aforementioned cytokines. These are proteins that trigger the production of more inflammatory mediators, such as C-reactive protein (CRP). CRP is just one inflammatory marker that doctors use to measure the body's inflammatory state. If there is inflammation anywhere in the body, CRP typically increases. The CRP level rises in cases of chronic infection, elevated blood sugar (insulin resistance), and in overweight and obese people, especially among those with increased belly fat. Elevated CRP is also associated with an increased risk of both heart attack and stroke.

When the body produces more inflammatory mediators, such as CRP, this in turn sparks chronic systemic inflammation. Essentially, the more fat you have (particularly belly fat), the more inflammation you suffer.

Most people think of fat tissue as inactive, but that is far from the truth. Fatty tissue or fat storage areas, such as belly fat, are active endocrine organs that produce numerous types of hormones, such as resistin (which increases insulin resistance), leptin (which decreases appetite), and adiponectin (which improves insulin sensitivity and helps to lower blood sugar). The more fat cells, the more estrogen, cortisol, and testosterone your body produces. This is one of the reasons obese men typically develop breasts and obese women often grow hair on their face. Their fat cells are manufacturing more estrogen and testosterone, respectively.

Going Low Glycemic

A recent study of the Dutch population found that by lowering the glycemic index value of overall food intake by an average of ten points, participants decreased their CRP levels by 29 percent. Participants who continued on a low-glycemic diet also had higher levels of good cholesterol, improved insulin sensitivity, and reduced chronic inflammation—all of which indicated a decrease in risk of metabolic syndrome and cardiovascular disease.[2]

When your fatty tissues spew out all these hormones—most likely raising your estrogen, testosterone, and cortisol levels—and produce tremendous inflammation in your body, the result is weight gain. Your extra toxic belly fat then sets the stage for type 2 diabetes, heart disease, stroke, cancer, and a host of other diseases. That's because belly fat is like those Southwestern wildfires I mentioned earlier. It spreads throughout your body and inflames your cardiovascular system, which causes the production of plaque in your arteries and inflammation in the brain. This can even potentially lead to Alzheimer's disease.

THE PROOF IS IN THE FAT

Several studies show the parallels between inflammation and fat. One study found that inflammation increased more than 50 percent in obese women whose fat was primarily in their hips and thighs. Among women with abdominal obesity, that number rose to a staggering 400 percent.[3]

A quick review may help you better understand the

fat-inflammation connection. Every pound of stored fat requires about a mile's worth of blood vessels to sustain itself. In order to exist, fat cells secrete hormonelike substances to increase blood vessel growth. These blood vessels are supposed to nourish and feed accumulated fat. However, when the blood vessel growth cannot keep up with expanding fat, the fat cells become deprived of oxygen. These oxygen-deprived cells then release more inflammatory mediators to trigger more blood vessel growth…and on it goes. The wildfire spreads, made worse when the spark comes from belly fat, the most flammable source.

Other studies underscore the fact that inflammation not only *prepares* the body for adding additional fat but also even *precedes* this process. Two studies, the Atherosclerosis Risk in Communities Study and the Healthy Women Study, found higher concentrations of CRP and fibrinogen before weight gain occurred.[4] (Fibrinogen is a protein in the blood that, when elevated, can lead to blood clots or an increased risk of heart attacks and strokes.) Further research from Sweden showed that the higher the number of elevated inflammatory proteins, the greater the chances of weight gain.[5] Prior to these reports, experts assumed that obese people had higher levels of inflammatory proteins because of the cytokines their fatty tissues secreted. In other words, doctors thought that obese individuals continued to deal with greater inflammation because they were obese. Instead these studies proved the other way was equally true: the higher the inflammatory proteins, the greater the odds of weight gain.

Without a doubt, fat deposited in the abdominal area leads to the greatest amount of inflammation. Conversely, when you decrease your body's inflammatory response, you will also lower your weight and your waist size. Given this situation, it is helpful to know which foods can trigger inflammation and which ones help control it.

A DEADLY BY-PRODUCT OF THE WESTERN DIET: INFLAMMATION

One of the biggest problems with our modern, high-fat, highly processed, high-sugar, high-grain (such as wheat and corn), high-sodium diets is that it has thrown off the balance in our bodies between inflammatory and anti-inflammatory chemicals called *prostaglandins*. Normally inflammation is a good thing that works to repair an injury or fight off infection in the body. It puts the immune system on high alert to attack invading bacteria or viruses to rid our body of these intruders, or in the case of an injury, it rushes white blood cells to the cut, scrape, sprain, or broken bone to remove the damaged cells or attack infections to facilitate healing. This is the good side of inflammation and an extremely important function of the immune system's small agents. When our bodies are in such an emergency, there is a complicated process through which more pro-inflammatory prostaglandins are created than anti-inflammatory ones, and the immune system responds to the sounding of this alarm. When the crisis is over, the balance swings in the anti-inflammatory direction and eventually balances out again.

If you look at this process in a grossly simplified sense, you will see that prostaglandins are produced from the foods we eat in an ongoing cycle, and each of the foods we eat has either a pro-inflammatory tendency or an anti-inflammatory one. Fatty acids are at the center of this. Omega-6 fatty acids are "friendly" to the creation of pro-inflammatory prostaglandins, and omega-3 fatty acids are "friendly" to the creation of anti-inflammatory prostaglandins. A more natural, Mediterranean-type diet will have a balance of pro- and anti-inflammatory-friendly foods; however, our modern high-fat, high-sodium, high-sugar, highly processed Western diet throws that balance off in favor of the production of pro-inflammatory prostaglandins.

Experts tell us that our typical US diet has doubled the amount of omega-6 fatty acids we consume since 1940 as we have shifted more and more away from fruits and vegetables to grain-based foods and the oils produced from them. In fact, we eat about twenty times more omega-6s than we do the anti-inflammatory omega-3s. Most of the animals we obtain food from today are also grain fed, so most of our meats, eggs, and dairy products are higher in omega-6s than they were a century ago. Also, as most of the fish in our stores are now farm raised, they are fed a diet of cereal grains instead of the algae and smaller fish they would live on in the wild, so even our fish are more sources of omega-6s than they used to be. Noting all of this, it is not hard to see why diseases caused by chronic systematic inflammation have grown to be such a problem in the Western world today.

Furthermore, essential fatty acids (EFAs) such as omega-3 and omega-6 cannot be manufactured in the body and must be consumed either through diet or supplements. EFAs help the body repair and create new cells. In addition to reducing inflammation, omega-3 fatty acids can actually create special roadblocks in the body, making it harder for cancer cells to migrate from a primary tumor to start new colonies. Cancers that remain localized in one place are much easier to treat than those that metastasize (spread throughout the body).[6]

Because of the high omega-6 content of our diets, our bodies find more material for pro- than anti-inflammatory prostaglandins. Over time the natural, ongoing creation of prostaglandins will tip the balance toward systematic inflammation as more pro-inflammatory prostaglandins are produced than anti-inflammatory ones. Despite the absence of an actual emergency, this imbalance still sets off alarms calling for inflammation, and the immune system will respond accordingly. However, with no actual threat present, the immune system will start attacking things it normally wouldn't. This immune hypersensitivity can lead to a glut of problems ranging from simple allergies and weight gain to cancer, Alzheimer's disease, cardiovascular disease, diabetes, arthritis, asthma, prostate problems, and autoimmune diseases.

Many of these happen because as the immune system stays on high alert longer than it should, its agents begin to fatigue and make bad decisions, possibly leading to autoimmune disease or not destroying mutated cells, leading to cancer formation with more frequency. This can easily give way to cancer getting a foothold it won't easily relinquish.

Omega-3 fatty acids are clearly incredibly beneficial. Here are some omega-3 foods to include in your diet: flaxseeds and flaxseed oil, chia seeds, fish (salmon, sardines, halibut, tongol tuna, herring, and cod), and fish oil. Obviously it's important to know which fats to eat and which ones to avoid when it comes to preventing those harmful prostaglandins I mentioned above.

So, while using an understanding of the Mediterranean diet as a foundation, within that framework you should also look at how pro-inflammatory or anti-inflammatory the foods you eat are as well. If you are having problems with allergies, joint pains, muscle aches, or the like, by eating more anti-inflammatory foods than pro-inflammatory ones, you can tip your balance back in the right direction.

One way to check your degree of inflammation is to have a C-reactive protein blood test. C-reactive protein is a promoter of inflammation and also a blood marker of systemic inflammation. Once you reach forty years of age, annual CRP testing is a great idea for checking the anti-inflammatory effectiveness of your diet. Men should aim for a CRP less than 1.0, while women should aim for a CRP less than 1.5.

FOODS THAT TRIGGER INFLAMMATION

Bad fats

Unfortunately, the standard American diet swings the balance toward excessive amounts of bad prostaglandins. This can increase inflammation and constrict blood vessels, setting the stage for hypertension, heart disease, heart attack, stroke, weight gain, and obesity, and diabetes.

Just Say No

Aleve and ibuprofen may seem like quick, easy, and affordable solutions for reducing inflammation. The same is true for various steroids (prednisone, cortisone, and Medrol) and nonsteroidal anti-inflammatory drugs. However, keep in mind that when used long term, all of these come with a potentially serious cost, such as the increased likelihood of heart attacks, stroke, and other ailments.

While defenders of the dietary status quo poke fun at health advocates or ridicule them as the "food police," the truth is that there are dangers in the types of fats we consume. The main types that trigger inflammation are trans fats, hydrogenated fats, and partially hydrogenated fats. These are generally found in margarines, shortenings, hydrogenated oils, and most baked goods. They are especially prevalent in cake icing, many commercial peanut butters, chips, crackers, cookies, and any foods that list hydrogenated or partially hydrogenated oils on the label. Fried foods—especially those that are deep-fried (e.g., fried chicken, french fries, fried fish)—also increase inflammation. You should also avoid excessive intake of saturated fats, which are found primarily in red meat, pork, processed meats, butter, whole milk, cheese, and poultry skins. All increase your chances of inflammation.

So do omega-6 fats, which are found in vegetable oils such as safflower, corn, soy, sunflower, and cottonseed oils. Most salad dressings, sauces, and gravies contain these inflammatory oils. Their labels will usually list "linoleic acid," "polyunsaturated, or "omega-6."

Top Ten Foods With Trans Fats

- Butter substitutes—margarine, shortening, and other non-butter spreads contain large amounts of trans fat.

- Packaged foods—cake mixes, pancake mixes, etc. All have several grams of trans fat per serving.

- Soups—Ramen noodles and soup cups contain high levels of trans fat.

- Fast food—fries, chicken strips, and other deep-fried foods are fried in hydrogenated oil.

- Frozen food—frozen pies, waffles, pizzas, and fish sticks contain trans fat.

- Baked goods—more trans fats are used in baked products (doughnuts, cookies, cakes, etc.) from your supermarket bakery than any other foods.

- Chips and crackers—anything fried or buttery has trans fat. Even reduced-fat brands can still have trans fat.

- Breakfast foods—most cereals and energy bars, even those that claim to be healthy, are highly processed and contain trans fats.

- Cookies and candy—a chocolate bar or cookie is likely to have more trans fat than gummy bears, so read labels.

- Toppings, flavorings, dips, and gravies—nondairy creamers and flavored coffees, whipped toppings, bean

dip, gravy mixes, and salad dressings contain a lot of
trans fat.[7]

Corn-fed beef

Corn-fed beef significantly increases inflammation, which is why you should search for "organic" or
"grass fed" designations on cuts of steak, hamburger,
and other meats. What difference does it make? Grass-
fed cattle have approximately six to eight times less fat
than grain-fed cattle, as well as two to six times more
omega-3 fats. These omega-3s decrease inflammation.
This is because the grass the livestock eat typically contains omega-3 fats that are eventually stored in their
flesh. Most livestock today are grain fed—usually corn.
This increases the omega-6 oils, overall fat, and saturated fats. Both fats are inflammatory, which means
that while you enjoy your hamburger or steak, you may
be inflaming your body.

By the way, chickens are fed similar grain as livestock. Feeding poultry a grain-based diet causes
chickens, as well as their eggs, to be loaded with pro-
inflammatory fats.

Foods high in arachidonic acid

Both saturated fats and omega-6 fats can convert to
arachidonic acid. Since this acid is a building block for
bad prostaglandins, it is wise to limit consumption of
this inflammatory fat. Foods rich in arachidonic acid
include fatty cuts of red meat and pork, egg yolks, high-
fat dairy products, shellfish, and organ meats.

The problem arises especially in men who can easily

consume a pound or two of steak, three to four eggs, a pint of ice cream, half a pound of cheese, a few table-spoons of butter, and a quart of whole milk daily. While periodically eating small portions (3 to 6 ounces) of lean, organic red meat is acceptable, eating mammoth-sized steaks or hamburger every day is a recipe for inflammatory disaster. When you eat large amounts of foods rich in arachidonic acid, your body increases its production of enzymes to break down the acid. This produces leukotriene B4 and other inflammatory mediators that can cause even more chronic inflammation.

Sugars

All sugars fan the fire inflammation in the body. They also weaken the immune system. Just 100 grams of sugar (the equivalent of three sodas) can weaken your immune system for five hours by as much as 50 percent. Excess sugar intake increases the production of arachidonic acid, which encourages cancer to develop and spread, encourages inflammation in the arteries leading to heart disease, and encourages inflammation in the joints leading to arthritis. It also accelerates aging. Women, the more inflammation that exists in your body, the faster you will age and the more wrinkles and sagging skin you will develop. Try keeping that in mind the next time you reach for a soda, dessert, or white bread.

Wheat

Excess wheat consumption is also very inflammatory. Until fifty years ago wheat had only modestly changed over the centuries since biblical times. However, modern wheat strains have been hybridized, crossbred, and genetically altered by agricultural scientists in order to increase crop production.[8]

Modern strains of wheat have a higher quantity of genes for gluten proteins that are associated with celiac disease.[9] Modern wheat contains a starch called amylopectin A that raises blood sugar levels more than virtually any other carbohydrate.[10]

Cardiologist William Davis, author of the book *Wheat Belly*, takes his patients off of all wheat and corn starch. Many Americans have what Dr. Davis calls a "wheat belly," and he associates this with high cholesterol, high triglycerides, hypertension, elevated blood sugar, diabetes, and obesity.

In addition, wheat is an appetite stimulant, making you want more and more food.[11] It's also considered addictive. Approximately 30 percent of all people who stop eating wheat products experience withdrawal symptoms such as extreme fatigue, mental fog, irritability, inability to function at work, and depression.[12]

FOODS THAT CONTROL INFLAMMATION

Good fats

Just as bad fats are a source of inflammation, good fats are the best fire extinguishers. Omega-3 fats from cold-water fish, wild fish instead of farm-raised fish, or high-quality omega-3 supplements are the best anti-inflammatory oils. Flaxseeds, chia seeds, hemp seeds, and Salba seeds are also good sources of omega-3 fats. Unfortunately the standard American diet is low in omega-3 fats and high in the inflammatory omega-6 fats.

The recommended ratio of omega-6 fats to omega-3 fats should be four to one. However, most Americans consume these in a ratio closer to twenty to one.

Fishy Tip

When shopping for a great source of omega-3 fats to reduce inflammation, keep in mind that all salmon from Alaska is wild, whereas Atlantic salmon is typically farmed. Just because a grocery store or restaurant labels its salmon "wild" doesn't necessarily mean it is. Farmed fish makes up 90 percent of this country's salmon sales, so do your homework to make sure you can trust certain brands, supermarkets, or eating establishments.[13]

Another good fat that helps decrease inflammation is gamma-linolenic acid, or GLA. Found in borage oil, black currant seed oil, and evening primrose oil, GLA is classified as an omega-6 oil, but it behaves more like an omega-3. Other good fats include the omega-9 family of fats; among them are olive oil, almonds, avocados, macadamia nuts, pecans, cashews, sunflower seeds, pumpkin seeds, and avocados. Walnuts, flaxseeds, and chia seeds are also good anti-inflammatory fats.

Increase fruits and vegetables

With the exception of potatoes and corn, almost all vegetables will help with inflammation. I recommend eating many different vegetables with a diversity of color—and choosing organic. Be aware that some vegetables classified as "nightshades" may trigger inflammation in some individuals, especially those with arthritis. Examples of nightshades are tomatoes, potatoes,

peppers, and eggplants. If after eating nightshade vegetables you experience joint aches, swelling, or redness;
rashes; or increased joint aches, you should probably
limit or avoid one or more of the nightshade vegetables.
Sometimes the inflammation from eating these vegetables occurs within a day or two. For other individuals it
may occur a few hours after consumption. If you suspect
nightshades are causing inflammation, refer to www
.worldhealth.net to find a physician experienced in diag-
nosing and treating food sensitivities.

When Activity Itches

For most people food allergy symptoms arrive shortly (if not
immediately) after consuming a particular food with allergens.
However, for a small segment of the population, such a reaction is
conditional on physical activity. Those who have physical-activity-
induced food allergies only detect it if they eat a certain food or foods
and then work out. As their body temperature increases, symptoms
such as itching, light-headedness, hives, asthma, or anaphylaxis can
appear. The remedy is as easy as not eating for at least two hours
before an activity session.

Some fruits and vegetables are particularly helpful in
calming inflammation. Onions, apples, red grapes, and
red wine all contain quercetin, a powerful antioxidant
that helps quench inflammation. Garlic, ginger, and
rosemary sprigs have anti-inflammatory properties. So
does curry powder, which contains curcumin, a highly
anti-inflammatory spice. In addition, pineapple contains bromelain, an enzyme that decreases inflammation. The herb Boswellia also decreases inflammation.

(For information on other foods that decrease inflammation, see my book *The Seven Pillars of Health*.)

A sensible program like I recommend on the Rapid Waist Reduction Diet succeeds because it includes anti-inflammatory foods, including plenty of fruits and vegetables. It also helps users practice portion control, limits bad fats, and encourages the consumption of healthy fats. Essentially, when you learn how to substitute good fats for inflammatory fats; replace high-glycemic, refined carbohydrates with low-glycemic, high-fiber ones; and eat smaller portions of lean, organic, free-range meats in place of high-fat, grain-fed varieties, you dramatically decrease inflammation. Limiting or avoiding sugar, juices, sodas, desserts, and sugary coffees can also help quench these fires.

THE ANTI-INFLAMMATORY DIET: TAKING THE MEDITERRANEAN DIET TO THE NEXT LEVEL

So then, how do you escape this systematic inflammation that is causing so many people so many health problems? First of all, you adopt the Mediterranean diet as the foundation for your day-in, day-out meal planning.

Then, within that framework, balance your pro-inflammatory and anti-inflammatory foods as your body and your CRP tests indicate that you should. This will, of course, initially probably mean adding more anti-inflammatory foods and avoiding the pro-inflammatory ones for a time.

I have organized the following two lists of foods for

you to consider adding or subtracting from your diet as your level of systematic inflammation demands.

TOP ANTI-INFLAMMATORY FOODS (ALWAYS CHOOSE ORGANIC WHEN POSSIBLE)	
Fruit	Raspberries, acerola (West Indian) cherries, guava, strawberries, cantaloupe, lemons/limes, rhubarb, kumquat, pink grapefruit, mulberries, blueberries, blackberries
Vegetables	Chili peppers, onions (including scallions and leeks), spinach, greens (including kale, collards, and turnip and mustard greens), sweet potatoes, carrots, garlic
Legumes	Lentils, green beans, peas
Egg Products	Liquid eggs, egg whites (may use one organic or free-range egg yolk with three egg whites)
Dairy (use with caution)	Cottage cheese (low fat and nonfat), nonfat cream cheese, plain low-fat Greek yogurt or vanilla Greek yogurt (add fresh fruit if desired) (Limit dairy to 4–6 oz. every three to four days)
Fish	Herring, mackerel (not king), wild salmon (not farmed; Alaskan preferred), rainbow trout, sardines, anchovies
Poultry	Goose, duck, free-range organic chicken and turkey (white meat preferred, skins removed) (3–6 oz. once or twice a day)
Meat	Eye of round (beef), flank steak, sirloin tip, skirt steak, pork tenderloin (free range preferred, extra lean or lean) (Limit to 3–6 oz. two times a week)
Cereal	Steel-cut oatmeal, oat bran
Fats/Oils	Safflower oil (high oleic), hazelnut oil, olive oil, avocado oil, almond oil, apricot kernel oil

Nuts/Seeds	Brazil nuts, macadamia nuts, hazelnuts, pecans, almonds, hickory nuts, cashews (best raw)
Herbs/Spices	Garlic, onion, cayenne, ginger, turmeric, chili peppers, chili powder, curry powder, rosemary, ginger, boswellia
Sweeteners	Stevia, tagatose, coconut palm sugar
Beverages	Tomato juice, black or green tea, club soda/seltzer, herbal tea, spring water
Starches	Sweet potatoes, new potatoes, millet bread, brown and wild rice, brown rice pasta, and legumes (see above for approved legumes)

INFLAMMATORY FOODS TO LIMIT OR AVOID	
Fruit	Mango, banana, dried apricots, dried apples, dried dates, canned fruits, raisins
Vegetables	Corn, white potatoes, french fries
Legumes	Baked beans, fava beans (boiled), canned beans
Egg Products	Duck eggs, goose eggs, hard-boiled eggs, egg yolks
Cheeses	Brick cheese, cheddar cheese, Colby cheese, cream cheese (normal and reduced fat)
Dairy	Fruited yogurt, ice cream, butter
Fish	Farmed salmon
Poultry	Turkey (dark meat), Cornish game hen, chicken giblets, chicken liver
Meat	Bacon, veal loin, veal kidney, beef lung, beef kidney, beef heart, beef brain, pork chitterlings, lamb rib chops, turkey breast with skin, turkey wing with skin, all processed meats

Breads	Hot dog/hamburger buns, English muffins, kaiser rolls, bagels, french bread, Vienna bread, blueberry muffins, oat bran muffins
Cereal	Grape-Nuts, Crispix, Corn Chex, Just Right, Rice Chex, corn flakes, Rise Krispies, Raisin Bran, shredded wheat
Pasta/Grain	White rice, lasagna noodles, macaroni elbows, regular pasta, all corn products except corn on the cob or frozen corn (non-GMO)
Fats/Oils	Margarine, wheat germ oil, sunflower oil, poppy seed oil, grape seed oil, safflower oil, cottonseed oil, palm kernel oil, corn oil
Nuts/Seeds	Poppy seeds, walnuts, pine nuts, sunflower seeds
Sweeteners	Honey, brown sugar, white sugar, corn syrup, powdered sugar
Crackers/ Chips/Cookies	Corn chips, pretzels, graham crackers, saltines, vanilla wafers
Desserts	Sweetened condensed milk, angel food cake, chocolate and vanilla cake with frosting, chocolate chips, heavy whipping cream, ice cream, fruit leather snacks (Most all desserts are made with sugar.)
Candy	Hershey Kisses, jelly beans, Twix, Almond Joy, milk chocolate bars, Snickers
Beverages	Milk, Gatorade, pineapple juice, orange juice, cranberry juice, lemonade, sodas, sugar-laden soft drinks

These are not complete lists by any means—just some of the more likely "suspects" to watch out for and some of the more helpful helpers to work into your diet. As you read these now, some of them will jump out at you as things you like and need, but you don't have as much of them in your diet as you probably should. Others are the foods that it is time to change your habits about and say good-bye to. The thing to remember is that you have a choice about what you put in your mouth, and now that you have a little more knowledge about these foods, you can begin making healthier diet choices concerning them.

If you have no health problems or obesity, avoiding the inflammatory foods on the previous pages is a good general guideline. Because your health is good, you have a little more freedom than someone who is struggling with his or her health or weight. You may eat some of the inflammatory foods listed, but I highly recommend you use moderation when consuming them.

If you have health problems or obesity, then in addition to understanding the anti-inflammatory and inflammatory food lists on the previous pages, I advise you to adhere to the following anti-inflammatory diet exactly as directed below and avoid all inflammatory foods. Once your health conditions clear up or you are able to maintain a healthy weight, you can ease up on the following guidelines, but again use moderation whenever eating inflammatory foods.

DR. COLBERT'S ANTI-INFLAMMATORY DIET *(ALWAYS CHOOSE ORGANIC WHEN POSSIBLE.)*	
Vegetables	Steam, stir fry, or cook under low heat Best cooked with olive oil, macadamia nut oil, or coconut oil Vegetable soups, non-cream-based, homemade is best; you may add some organic meat Juice your own vegetable juice; avoid store-bought juices, which are high in sodium.
Animal proteins (meat)	3.5 oz. once or twice a day for women; 6 oz. once or twice a day for men Wild salmon, sardines, anchovies, tongol tuna, turkey (skin removed), free-range chicken (skin removed), eggs (omega-3 eggs as well), bison, or extra-lean beef When grilling, slice meat into thin slices; marinate in red wine, pomegranate juice, cherry juice, or curry sauce. Remove all char from meat. Be cautious with egg yolks, keeping to a maximum of once or twice a week. You can combine one yolk with two to three egg whites. Lean beef and red meat, limit consumption to one to two servings a week
Fruits	Berries, Granny Smith apples, lemon, or lime Juicing these fruits is acceptable, but avoid store-bought juices, which are high in sugar.
Nuts and seeds	All raw nuts and seeds
Salads	Use 1-calorie-per-spray salad spritzers.
Dairy	Consume with caution; limit to every three to four days. See beverages below for alternatives to drinking cow's milk. Low-fat dairy without sugar such as Greek yogurt and low-fat cottage cheese

Starches	Sweet potatoes, new potatoes, brown/wild rice, millet bread, brown rice pasta, beans, peas, legumes, and lentils Use moderation when choosing starches, at most only one serving per meal.
Beverages	Alkaline water or sparkling water; may add lemon or lime Green, black, or white tea; may add lemon or lime Coffee Low-fat coconut milk or almond milk in place of cow's milk No sugar; use stevia or other sugar substitutes mentioned in this book to sweeten No cream; use low-fat coconut milk

FOODS TO AVOID ON DR. COLBERT'S ANTI-INFLAMMATORY DIET

- Avoid all gluten (wheat, barley, rye, spelt); this includes all products made with these grains, including bread, pasta, crackers, bagels, pretzels, most cereals, etc. Go to www.celiacsociety.com for gluten-free foods.

- Inflammatory animal proteins such as shellfish, pork, lamb, veal, and organ meats

- Sugar

- Fried foods

- Processed foods

- High glycemic foods such as white rice, instant potatoes, etc.

Be sure to rotate your vegetables and meats every four days. Do not eat the same food every day. For example, one day eat chicken, the next day eat turkey, the next day eat salmon, and so on.

Chapter 3

CULPRIT #2: CARBS— ESPECIALLY WHEAT

CARBS. AMERICANS LOVE them. And we need them. The truth is, certain carbohydrates are critical for good health. When combined with the correct portions of fats and proteins, good carbs give you energy, calm your mood, keep you full and satisfied by turning off hunger, and assist in weight loss. They also help you to enjoy meals and snacks, enable you to handle stress better, allow you to sleep more soundly, improve your bowel function, and give you an overall feeling of well-being.

However, as with so many things in the land of excess, we have fallen in love with the wrong kind of carbs. It is easy to find bad carbs—they're everywhere! In the same way that restaurants have taken unhealthy portions to new heights, manufacturers have undermined the purpose of healthy food. Manufacturers have taken the best of nature—fruits, vegetables, potatoes, sugarcane, corn, wheat, rice, and other grains—and processed and refined them by milling, pressing, squeezing, cooking, and separating whole foods into parts. Their procedures turn natural foods into man-made nightmares. Instead of fruit, we get processed, pasteurized juice, jams, pastries, and the like. Instead of sugarcane and corn, we end up with white sugar and sodas containing fattening, high-fructose corn syrup. Instead of whole-wheat bread, we get white bread, crackers, pasta, highly processed cereals, buns, bagels, pretzels, cakes, or muffins. And instead of brown rice or wild rice, we get white rice and rice cakes.

To help my patients lose weight I first have them give up all wheat and corn products for a season or until they reduce their belly fat. Then once they reach their goal waist measurement or weight, if they can practice moderation, I add back small servings for breakfast or lunch but not dinner.

LOSE THE WHEAT, LOSE THE WEIGHT

According to renowned cardiologist William Davis, MD, foods made with wheat or containing wheat are the number one reason Americans are fat. He goes as far as to say, "Overly enthusiastic wheat consumption is the *main* cause of the obesity and diabetes crisis in the United States."[1] This is why he feels low-carb diets are among the most successful diets. Cut carbs, and you will automatically cut wheat. Because wheat dominates the diets of most modern adults (the average American consumes 133 pounds of wheat per year[2]), removing wheat removes the biggest problem. According to Dr. Davis:

> It makes perfect sense: If you eliminate foods that trigger exaggerated blood sugar and insulin responses, you eliminate the cycle of hunger and momentary satiety, you eliminate the dietary

source of addictive exorphins, you are more satisfied with *less*. Excess weight dissolves and you
revert back to physiologically appropriate weight.
You lose the peculiar and unsightly ring around
your abdomen: Kiss your wheat belly goodbye.[3]

BAD HABITS

With all the bad carbs at our disposal, it's easy to see
why in recent years all carbohydrates have received a
bad rap. I have met countless individuals who, during
their initial appointments with me, preached about the
detriments of all carbs because that's what they had
learned from past dieting experiences. They had climbed
on board the high-protein diet train and weren't about
to get off—even though such regimens had damaged
their health. At times it was downright funny how ada-
mantly they swore off carbs, as if touching them would
instantly add a pound or two. The problem was, they
couldn't sustain the no-carb approach for long. That is
why they were in my office, weighing more than before
starting their diet.

The National Institutes of Health recommends that
45 to 65 percent of our daily energy intake come from
carbohydrates, with 25 to 35 percent of energy coming
from fats and only 15 to 35 percent from proteins.[4] The
American Diabetes Association also recommends 45
to 60 grams of carbohydrates in each meal, preferably
from healthy whole grains. I believe this is too many
carbohydrates and too much grain. I believe excessive
carbohydrates and grains—especially wheat and corn
products—are one of the main reasons for our obesity

epidemic. I typically recommend about 50 percent of daily calories come from low-glycemic carbohydrates, 20 percent from plant and lean animal proteins, and 25 to 30 percent from healthy fats.

Have you ever wondered why there aren't more restaurants and fast-food chains touting natural carbs, such as steel-cut oats, whole fruits, broccoli, asparagus, beans, peas, or legumes? First, because these carbs are more filling—meaning customers rarely overeat them and are less likely to purchase other items on the menu. Second, these types of carbs do not have as long a shelf life—which should make you wonder what exactly is being put in the bad carbs to make them last so long.

The Tortoise and the Hare

Many people are familiar with the old story about the tortoise and the hare. The hare races ahead but fails to reach the finish line, while the slow but steady tortoise eventually passes him and wins the race. When it comes to how your body processes carbohydrates, the race that takes place within you is reminiscent of this classic fable. I've used these familiar characters to identify two main types of carbohydrates: "tortoise carbs" and "hare carbs."

Before going further, I should explain that I am not talking about simple carbs vs. complex carbs, which are two common categories of carbs. Instead I will call low-glycemic carbs the "tortoise" and high-glycemic carbs the "hare."

Unfortunately, most of the carbohydrates overweight and obese people consume are not the kinds that assist with weight loss. Instead they are high-glycemic "hare carbs," which cause the blood sugar to rise rapidly. As I have already alluded to, this starts a chain of events that trap people in a fat-storage mode and prevent them from losing weight. The underlying cycle of hare carbs is obvious enough: the faster you absorb the carbs, the higher your insulin level rises, the more weight you gain, and the more diseases you develop. You become literally programmed for weight gain.

Welcome to the dark side of carbohydrates, where restaurant menus, grocery-store shelves, and home pantries overflow with highly processed, high-glycemic carbs. This romance with processed foods—such as breads, potatoes, corn starch, and other grains—is one of the main reasons we see obesity increasing at alarming rates. Yet it doesn't have to be this way.

Remember, even if breads at the supermarket are called whole-grain breads, they still contain amylopectin A, which usually spikes the blood sugar, programming the body for fat storage and weight gain. Therefore if my patients request bread, I recommend that they have small amounts of millet bread in the morning or at lunch. It contains no wheat. I find that it tastes better when toasted. You can find millet bread in many health food stores or online. However, if weight loss stalls, I have my patients stop eating millet bread.

CARBOHYDRATE AND SUGAR ADDICTS

When people crave highly processed carbohydrates, they are usually craving sugars. More often than not they are hooked on sugar. The digestive system quickly turns those highly processed carbs into sugar, which is rapidly absorbed into the bloodstream. This, in turn, spikes insulin, which drives the sugar into the cells and tissues. In only a few hours, when the cells in the hypothalamus sense inadequate sugar, appetite returns as the brain communicates that it needs a new "fix."

If you think I am going overboard with the drug addiction analogy, here's proof that I am not: Sugar and highly processed carbs release natural opioids in the brain. Your brain has opioid receptors. The phrase "runner's high" gets its name from the euphoric sensation that occurs when physical activity stimulates the brain to form endorphins. These neurotransmitters are similar in molecular structure to morphine, though much milder. They activate the brain's pleasure center.

Like exercise, sugars and the gluten in wheat are also able to trigger the release of such endorphins and gluteomorphins—which is why we call the result a "sugar high" or "sugar rush." Most people are unconsciously stimulating the pleasure centers in their brains by having a hit of sugar, bread, muffin, bagel, doughnut, soda, or something similar. This is proof of how easy it is to become a sugar or carbohydrate addict; we are naturally programmed this way.

This opioid effect—and our natural inclination for it—has even been verified in infants. At Johns Hopkins University, researchers studied one- to three-day-old infants to observe their response to sugar. These babies were each placed in a bassinet for five minutes. When they began to whimper or cry, researchers gave them either a small amount of sugar in water or just plain water. They discovered that those who received sugar water stopped crying, while the plain water did nothing to stop the crying.[5]

In addition to activating opioid receptors, sugar and highly processed carbs also have a physiologically calming affect because of the release of serotonin in the brain. When the brain's serotonin level increases after you have eaten sweets or a refined starch, within twenty to thirty minutes you typically experience significant emotional relief. This also suppresses your appetite, improves your mood, helps you relax, makes you sleep better, and contributes to an overall feeling of well-being. Meanwhile, your body is programmed to store fat, all the while craving the next intake of feel-good but highly processed carbs.

Tortoise Carbs

Over the years I have attended a few financial seminars on investing. At almost every one the financial expert used the tortoise-and-hare analogy to show how long-term investing always wins out in the end. Though some investors manage to beat the odds by playing the market for short-term gains, it is undoubtedly the slow and steady, "in it for the long haul" investors who wind up with greater earnings. Because of this, these instructors hardly spent any time talking about next year's hottest stocks. Instead they offered plenty of advice on how to find those stocks or mutual funds that were consistent winners.

When it comes to weight-loss success, "tortoise carbs" are like long-term investments. These are the carbohydrates that slowly raise the blood sugar and enable you to lose weight and prevent or reverse diseases. We have spent the first part of this chapter discussing the lousy effects of "hare carbs." I will spend the rest of the chapter on natural, unprocessed carbs that can keep you healthy.

For starters, low-glycemic tortoise carbs can be broken down into the following groups:

- Vegetables

- Fruits

- Starches, such as millet bread, brown rice pasta, steel-cut oatmeal, sweet potatoes, new potatoes, brown rice, and wild rice, in small quantities

- Dairy products, such as skim milk; low-fat, low-sugar yogurt; kefir; and low-fat cottage cheese

- Legumes, such as beans, peas, lentils, and peanuts

- Nuts and seeds (raw)

Even though most of these tortoise carbohydrates are healthy, it's still possible to choose the wrong types of starches and dairy or overeat low-glycemic starches, such as millet bread and brown rice pasta. For this reason, and because there are other ways carbohydrates stall weight-loss efforts, it's important to incorporate the glycemic index and glycemic load principles

I discuss in some of my other books, such as *Reversing Diabetes* and *Dr. Colbert's "I Can Do This" Diet*.

Is It a Hare or a Tortoise?

The faster your body digests a carbohydrate, the faster it raises your blood sugar—and the higher the glycemic index value of that carb. This is what makes a carb a hare rather than a tortoise. Yet how exactly can you differentiate between the two? Here are a few traits that will help distinguish between a tortoise and a hare.

Fat content. With the exception of seeds, nuts, and dairy, most tortoise carbohydrates are low in fat. Fats are not an inherent evil as some diets claim. In fact, adequate amounts of fats in a meal are absolutely essential for keeping you satisfied longer and slowing the rate at which carbohydrates are broken down and released into the bloodstream—which is why most low-fat diets fail. This doesn't give you the license to down a bag of Doritos or other highly processed, high-fat carbohydrates just to get your fat content. Obviously you sabotage your weight-loss efforts when you do this.

Fiber content. Generally, a higher fiber content of a food slows down the absorption of sugar, making the carb a tortoise.

Form of starch. Certain starches, such as potatoes, bread, pasta, and white rice, contain amylopectin, which is a complex carbohydrate that the body rapidly absorbs and that usually raises one's blood sugar. However, beans, peas, legumes, and sweet potatoes contain another complex carb called amylose, which is digested more slowly and raises the blood sugar in a slower fashion as well. However, caution is needed with whole-wheat products since 75 percent of the complex carb in wheat is amylopectin A and only 25 percent is amylose. Almost all corn products, such as cornmeal, corn pasta, and corn flakes, are digested rapidly and therefore are considered hare carbohydrates (with a high glycemic index value). Exceptions are corn on the cob and frozen corn, because they are digested more slowly and only gradually raise the blood sugar.

The ABCs of Amylopectin

In the human GI tract both amylopectin and amylase are digested by the enzyme amylase. Amylopectin is quickly converted to glucose, while amylase is more slowly converted to glucose, with some of it making its way to the colon undigested. So amylopectin (which makes up 75 percent of the complex carb in wheat) is the key culprit behind the increase in blood sugar caused by wheat.

To make matters worse, there are different forms of amylopectin, and wheat contains the most digestible form.

- Legumes have amylopectin C, the least digestible form.

- Bananas and potatoes contain amylopectin B, which is more quickly converted to glucose than the form in legumes but still resists digestion to some degree.

- Amylopectin A, the form contained in wheat products, is the most digestible form of amylopectin and could be regarded as a "supercarbohydrate."[6]

Ripeness. The riper the fruit, the faster it is absorbed. An example of this is the difference between yellow bananas and brown, spotted bananas. The latter raise the blood sugar much faster than regular yellow bananas since they are riper and have a higher sugar content.

Cooking. Most brown rice pasta can be either a tortoise carbohydrate or a hare carbohydrate, depending on how you cook it. If you cook it al dente, still leaving it firm, it is typically a tortoise carbohydrate and has a low glycemic index value. It's easy to overcook rice pasta, so keep a close eye on it until you get the hang of it. Also, thicker pasta noodles generally have a lower glycemic index value than thinner types of pasta (angel hair, thin spaghetti, etc.). Again, I don't recommend any wheat pasta products, even whole grain, since they have a higher glycemic load than many other carbohydrates.

Milling type. A finely ground grain is a hare carbohydrate and has a higher glycemic index value than coarsely ground grain, which has a higher fiber content and thus is a tortoise.

Protein content. The higher the protein content of a food, the more it helps prevent a rapid rise in blood sugar and makes the food more likely to be lower glycemic. Thus it is a tortoise carbohydrate.

THE LESS SUGAR, THE BETTER

We have already talked about the different types of carbohydrates; now let's briefly discuss sugar. Unfortunately, statistics show that Americans have become too familiar with this elemental substance. The average American consumes about 156 pounds of sugar a year![7] Let's put that into perspective: A single 12-ounce can of carbonated soda typically contains 8 to 10 teaspoons of sugar.[8] If you drink soft drinks throughout the day, you can see how this added sugar intake quickly adds up. And it's even worse for teenagers, who consume a daily average of 28 teaspoons a day, compared to 21 teaspoons for adults.[9]

National Sugar High

In the early 1980s roughly one in seven Americans was obese and almost 6 million were diabetic. In 2012 one in three adults were obese, and 26 million were diabetic, according to the CDC.[10]

Most everyone knows the foods that are high in sugar—desserts, sodas, candy, cookies, cakes, pies, doughnuts, etc. The general public is a little less knowledgeable about those starchy foods that, while not touted as high-sugar items, usually have high glycemic values. I cannot stress enough how important avoiding sugar is to losing weight and reducing your waist size. I realize that this isn't easy. As I mentioned earlier, sugar often triggers the release of endorphins, which gives us a sugar high—and acts like a drug, leading to cravings for more and more sugar.

The trouble is that eating sugar programs our body for weight gain. It also makes us more susceptible to insulin resistance, metabolic syndrome, type 2 diabetes, and heart disease. Excess sugar also triggers free-radical reactions in our bodies, leading to chronic disease, accelerated aging, and plaque formation in our arteries. Especially in diabetics, excess sugar can cause glycation, where sugar molecules react with protein molecules to cause wrinkled skin and damaged tissues. The bottom line is that—contrary to those images projected in TV advertisements—too much sugar does not produce a pretty face or body. Eat too much, and you will end up flabby and wrinkled.

Use Safe Sweeteners

For several years the dieting gimmick was (and to a degree still is) simply replacing these excess sugars with artificial sweeteners. There are plenty of sweeteners available, the most widely known being aspartame and sucralose. I do not recommend either one of these. (For detailed reasons on why neither of these work, see *The Seven Pillars of Health*.) There are, however, three natural sweeteners that are safe and low glycemic.

Unnaturally Sweet

Splenda, which is made by turning sugar into a chlorocarbon, is approximately six hundred times sweeter than sugar.[11]

Stevia

This is an herbal sweetener with no calories and a glycemic index value of zero. It is my favorite; I use the liquid form in my coffee and tea. In this form it is very sweet—approximately two hundred times sweeter than sugar. Because of this, you only need to use a tiny amount. Stevia is also available in granulated form. Products such as Truvia contain granulated stevia in convenient single-serving packets and can be found in most grocery stores. If powdered or liquid stevia tastes too sweet, I suggest trying the granulated form, which is more like the consistency and sweetness of sugar.

Agave Nectar and High-Fructose Corn Syrup

In spite of what you may have heard, agave nectar is not made from the sap of the agave plant but from the starch of the agave root bulb. The agave root contains starch—similar to that in corn or rice—and a complex carbohydrate called inulin, which is made up of fructose.

Similar to the way cornstarch is converted into high-fructose corn syrup (HFCS), agave starch goes through a chemical process that converts the starch into a fructose-rich syrup—anywhere from 70 percent fructose and higher, according to several agave nectar websites.

That means that the refined fructose in agave nectar is even more concentrated than the fructose in HFCS. For comparison, the HFCS used in sodas is 55 percent refined fructose.[12] For this reason I do not recommend using agave as an alternative to sugar, syrup, or other sweeteners.

Xylitol

A sugar alcohol, xylitol also has a very low glycemic index value. It also kills bacteria and prevents dental cavities. I have used xylitol as a nose drop to treat patients with sinus infections. It tastes just like sugar, with no aftertaste, and is a good substitute for sugar for cooking or baking. However, because it is a sugar alcohol, some individuals may experience bloating, gas, diarrhea, or other gastrointestinal issues when using xylitol in larger quantities. Because it is a natural sweetener and our bodies do produce it, I still recommend using it, but initially in very low doses to avoid any GI disturbance. Also, most xylitol comes from corncorbs and trees in China. If one is allergic to corn, avoid xylitol.

Chicory

Chicory is a natural sweetener that usually contains chicory root, which is a prebiotic food that may help improve your GI function by providing food for the beneficial bacterial in the GI tract. In addition to supporting your weight-loss efforts, chicory does not promote tooth decay. It is available at retail stores like Whole Foods and many health food stores. I find it a wonderful, natural alternative to sugar and harmful artificial sweeteners without the intense sweet aftertaste that deters some people from using stevia. (See Appendix B.)

Tagatose

Tagatose is a naturally occurring sugar or monosaccharide present in only small amounts in dairy products, fruits, and cacao. It has a texture very similar to white table sugar (sucrose) and is comparable in sweetness. Tagatose, however, contains only 38 percent of the calories of table sugar and has minimal affect on blood glucose and insulin levels. Table sugar has a glycemic index of 68, fructose has a glycemic index of 24, but tagatose has a very low glycemic index of 3. Tagatose does not spike the blood sugar or insulin levels and actually decreases blood glucose in the liver. Clinical studies have found that tagatose significantly decreases glucose levels among healthy individuals and individuals who are prediabetic, most type 2 diabetics, and even many type 1 diabetics. However, doctors should still monitor their diabetic patients' blood sugar closely when they start using tagatose.[13] (See Appendix B.)

Coconut sugar

Coconut sugar, or coconut palm sugar, is a sugar that is produced from the sap of flower buds from the coconut palm tree. Coconut sugar has been used for thousands of years as a sweetener in Southeast and South Asia. Coconut sugar tastes similar to brown sugar but has a slight taste of caramel. It consists mainly of sucrose and smaller amounts of glucose and fructose. Coconut sugar has a glycemic index of 35, which means it is low glycemic. As I stated above, table sugar has a glycemic index of 68, and fructose has a glycemic index of 24.

Coconut sugar contains vitamins, including vitamin B_{12}, B_2, B_3, and B_6, and is a good source of minerals, including potassium, magnesium, zinc, and iron. It also contains sixteen amino acids, including L-glutamine, which is the most abundant amino acid in coconut sugar.

Coconut sugar is becoming more popular among health food enthusiasts and diabetics. The lower glycemic index may mean that coconut sugar is safer for diabetics, but their blood sugar still needs to be closely monitored. I do believe that coconut sugar is a better choice that white table sugar; however, very small amounts need to be used. (See Appendix B.)

Chapter 4

YOUR WAISTLINE IS
YOUR LIFELINE

H AVE YOU EVER ridden the Kingda Ka at Six
Flags in New Jersey? At 456 feet it is taller
than the Statue of Liberty. Dropping 418 feet
and reaching speeds of 128 miles per hour, the nation's
fastest roller coaster promises riders jaw-dropping
excitement. Just behind it is northern Ohio's Top Thrill
Dragster, which stretches 420 feet into the air and hur-
tles along at 120 miles per hour. This Cedar Point ride
has a cousin: the Millennium Force, dropping 300 feet
of its 310-feet height and zipping along at 93 miles per
hour. Superman: The Escape at Six Flags Magic Mountain in Valencia, California, reaches 100 miles per hour
as it drops 328 feet.[1]

Dieting can be compared to a roller-coaster ride, with
one additional feature: instead of ending in a couple
minutes, it never lets up and makes life miserable when
it jerks you back up the weight-filled mountain. After a
while it becomes difficult to find another reason to continue. In nearly three decades of practicing medicine, I
have met countless numbers of overweight ex-dieters
who were stuck in self-defeating mental attitudes

toward weight loss. Their outlook sabotaged any hope of losing pounds.

Have you been battling a weight problem all of your life? No one has to tell you that many cases of disease are directly linked to obesity. Determine right now that, with God's help, you will get to your ideal weight and stay there. Perhaps you've been overweight for so long that you've given up. In the back of your mind you may even be thinking, "It's impossible for me to lose weight."

The truth is that your thinking is also your biggest obstacle to weight loss. If you want to lose weight but have been stuck on a dieting roller coaster, you can likely list 101 reasons *not to* diet. Who wants to embark on a boring, rigid, tasteless food regimen? At the same time, though, none of us want to be overweight or obese. Most people want to look good, feel good, and live a long, healthy life.

It's Your Life

Take a look at the top ten excuses for not dieting listed below. Do you see the potential for a downward spiral when you get stuck in this kind of thinking? It is a self-propelling trap. Most dieters become virtual excuse-makers, first blaming their circumstances and then themselves for their failures. Most reach a point where they either give in or see a doctor as a last resort.

Top Ten Excuses for Not Dieting

1. "I just can't resist my favorite foods."

2. "My social life is just too crazy."

3. "I don't have time to lose weight or plan meals."

4. "My family and friends won't support me."

5. "I don't have anyone to hold me accountable."

6. "It's too confusing to find which diet works for me."

7. "I travel too much."

8. "Dieting is too restrictive."

9. "It's too expensive to diet."

10. "I'm just too impatient to diet."[2]

The common problem I see among repeat dieters is that they focus on their weight instead of the simple lifestyle and dietary changes they need to make. Then, when their weight doesn't budge, they get discouraged and often stop the program all together. Or there is the other extreme, when people hit their target weight and abandon all reason, quickly sliding back into old eating patterns—the same ones that got them on the diet in the first place!

WHY DO YOU WANT TO LOSE WEIGHT?

It is great to set your mind to something and accept responsibility for your actions, whether looking at the past or toward the future. Yet such a radical shift in perspective can easily become just another mental pep talk that eventually fizzles out. What must accompany this change of heart is an underlying reason—one that comes straight from the heart. To switch to a can-do lifestyle, you need something that compels you from deep within.

Over the years I have observed that if your motive for losing weight is for any person other than yourself, the odds of failure are high. You should be doing this *for yourself*, to make you healthy, not to please someone else. Unfortunately too many women are tempted to lose weight for their spouse or boyfriend. Inevitably these are the women who find themselves back in the blame-shame-guilt cycle, particularly if this other person walks out of their life. I hate to sound cynical, but I have seen too many women do this and gradually regain their weight.

Many obese people are the same way. They have heard plenty of reasons from others why they should lose weight, yet they lack a personal driving force for *why* they should do it. If you are overweight and have never identified this reason, I urge you to do what I suggest to my obese patients: disrobe in front of a full-length mirror at home. Then analyze yourself from the front and back. Ask yourself: What are the main things that concern or bother me about being overweight or obese? Is it:

- The size of your hips, thighs, waist, or buttocks?

- The way your clothes fit?

- The way people treat or mistreat you?

- The embarrassing comments others make about you?

- Rejection from family members, friends, or coworkers?

- Being passed over for promotions because of your weight?

- Because your health is being affected by your weight?

- Because you have type 2 diabetes and do not want to develop the complications of diabetes?

Some people can answer these questions more easily by writing their thoughts in a journal. If that is the case, sit down and take the time to do it. This is an important exercise. If you are completely honest, the answers may change your life. As you come to grips with why you—and only you—want to lose weight and have decided to do so, you are ready to take responsibility for controlling your weight. Most individuals who have lost weight and kept it off did just that. Making this choice empowered them to lose weight by developing new, healthy habits. You may have unique reasons that only come by looking in the mirror, but the important thing is that you arrive in a new place of hope, determination, and purpose.

FACING THE TOUGH QUESTIONS

Will weight loss improve your marriage? You would think that the obvious answer is yes. However, after treating many overweight couples, I have often found that is not necessarily true. When one spouse loses weight and the other one does not, many times the spouse who has lost weight gets more attention from the opposite sex at work, out shopping, or while running errands. Some men and women have never had this kind of attention. It is flattering and enticing. Are you and your spouse prepared for possible feelings of jealousy, intimidation, and flattery? At the other extreme, some people have subconsciously gained weight to protect themselves from the pain of being rejected or from going through another painful relationship or breakup. Have you thought through how these issues affect your current and future health?

Also, will you be ready to purchase a new wardrobe in a few months? While the very thought of shopping excites most women, some men get physically ill at the notion of buying expensive new clothing. In addition, are you prepared for the possibility of a promotion or demotion at work? Yes, a leaner and trimmer image may be all you need for that promotion. Or it may spark jealousy from your boss, who reacts by moving you to another department. Understand that by losing weight, people will see you differently and treat you differently.

My point in asking these questions is not to plant fear or worry in your mind but to help you recognize that things will change when you lose weight—often drastically. I want you to be prepared to deal with these changes. Some patients who lose large amounts of weight ultimately need psychological counseling. To me that is a wonderful sign that they are accepting drastic changes and allowing others to help them walk through them. If you feel you need such guidance, don't hesitate to seek it out, maybe even before you start losing. The important thing is that you ask yourself these questions now so that you will not sabotage your weight loss later with wrong thoughts.

Also, examine the issue of timing, which often gets overlooked when people decide to embark on a life-changing journey. Earlier I listed ten common excuses for not dieting, but the truth is you only need one. It is important that you make sure the timing is right for you and that you have counted the cost before you start. Here's a statement that may surprise you: if you are in the midst of a major stressful time in your life such as a divorce, a life-threatening illness, a serious accident, a lawsuit, an IRS audit, a move, a job change, or some other major life event, *it is time to start.*

Before you question my sanity, hear me out. I realize that most diet books would tell you to forgo the diet until the major stress passes. However, it is in the midst of chaos that you want to find a lifestyle that can bring sanity, peace, assurance, and hope. Over the years I have found that when simple dietary and lifestyle principles are practiced regularly, they help you to manage stress and prevent stress eating.

WEIGHT-GAIN MENTALITY

Earlier I stated that your biggest obstacle for weight loss is your thinking. Most of my overweight and obese patients are stuck in what I call weight-gain mentality. They unknowingly have their mental channel tuned to it. As a result, they continue to attract more weight to themselves. I tell patients dealing with this problem that their autopilot is stuck on weight gain. You may have seen the same thing happening in your life. It is vital to remember that the ultimate success of any weight-loss program depends not on how much you eat but on what you think and believe.

The Bible repeatedly makes mention of this, often as the law of seedtime and harvest. Galatians 6:7 states, "Whatever a man sows, that he will also reap." In other words, if a farmer plants wheat, he will reap a harvest of wheat; if he plants corn, he will reap a harvest of corn. Elsewhere, Proverbs 23:7 says of a person that "as he thinks in his heart, so is he." This simply means that whatever you think about most, you will eventually become. Similarly Jesus says in Mark 11:24, "Whatever things you ask when you pray, believe that you receive them, and you will have them."

Since it is important that you believe you can achieve weight loss, it vital to speak affirmations of your desired weight, pants size, or dress size aloud throughout the day. Even if you weigh 250 pounds, you can state aloud that you see yourself weighing 140 pounds or wearing a size 8, or whatever pants or dress size you desire. Hebrews 11:1 defines faith as "the substance of things hoped for, the evidence of things not seen." Romans 4:17 speaks of calling those things that are not as though they are. So if you hope to weigh 140 pounds or wear a size 8 pair of jeans, start visualizing yourself at that weight and speak it aloud a few times a day.

Do not say, "I have to lose 100 pounds," or you will probably always have that many pounds to lose. Likewise, don't get in the habit of saying, "I'm planning on losing 50 pounds," or you will forever be *planning* to do that. Simply look at the picture of you at your desired weight and speak your desired weight aloud: "I see myself weighing _____ pounds," or "I weigh _____ pounds." (Fill in the blank.) Make that affirmation throughout the day, and as you follow through with your weight-loss program, you will naturally be attracted toward that desired weight, size, or image.

I have seen patients who struggled with weight for years do this, and they turned around and told me that losing weight became one of the easiest things they've ever done! I believe you will be making the same statement when you reach your ideal weight. This is not difficult. Start by making the decision to lose weight for yourself and no one else, and understand that you are the only one responsible for being overweight.

BURN OFF THAT BELLY FAT!

One of the main goals in reversing your risk of many diseases is to reduce your waist measurement. In fact, lowering waist size ranks higher than weight loss. As I've already explained, the abdominal region becomes a storehouse for toxic fat. For optimal health, a man should strive initially to get his waist measurement to less than 40 inches, while a woman should aim for an initial goal of less than 35 inches.

Along with specific diet and exercise programs, it is important to take certain nutritional supplements. Supplements can often pinpoint areas that regular eating or exercising cannot. Important supplements for carbohydrate metabolism include cinnamon, chromium, lipoic acid, B vitamins, and omega-3 fats. Since the refining process for most white breads, white rice, and other refined foods means they have lost most of their fiber and nutrient content, these foods lack many of the valuable nutrients for carbohydrate metabolism. Eating these nutrient-poor foods over the long term may eventually lead to nutrient deficiencies. That is why the supplements listed above, plus a good multivitamin, are all important.

OVERCOMING THE EPIDEMIC

Processed foods are taking a toll on the United States, whose residents have become addicted to sugars and highly refined carbohydrates. Any health practitioner, nutritionist, or dietician can draw a straight line between these habits and the obesity epidemic. Despite high levels of education and ever-increasing access to information via smartphones, the Internet, and other electronic tools, the average person is lost in the maze of information. Plodding along, stuck in lifelong familial and cultural habits, men and women alike can get easily locked into a lifestyle of eating zero-nutrition foods. After you read this, I hope you can see the connection between all these elements and the rise of obesity, which has reached epidemic levels.

Correcting the problem starts with your diet. Such everyday foods as white and wheat breads, crackers, bagels, pretzels, chips, pasta, white rice, potatoes, corn starch, instant oatmeal, most cereals, and sodas are not only part of the average American's diet, but they are also some of the main culprits behind developing insulin resistance. Trans fats, excessive saturated fats, and excessive omega-6 fats also contribute to insulin resistance and are equally common in salad dressings, fried foods, most dairy, processed meats and fatty cuts of meats, and sauces. Everywhere you look in America there are large portion sizes. You deserve a break today from this unhealthy glut of harmful substances. Pass the good health test by paying more attention to the fat, sugar, and sodium content of your diet. It will make a difference: just as the consequences of poor eating choices build over time, wise eating will bring long-term benefits. Just be patient!

The second main reason for our nation's epidemic of obesity is our lack of physical activity. We have become a society of couch potatoes. With age and inactivity we are losing valuable muscle mass. And because of our inactivity, we are developing a third problem: toxic belly fat, which increases our risk of many diseases.

These three elements—poor dietary choices (including large portion sizes), lack of exercise, and increasing belly fat—make up the vicious cycle that has locked millions of Americans into weight gain and increased risk of diseases. Many people have given up and are turning to fad diets, medications, and even lap-band surgery and other methods to help them lose weight. You don't have to do this! Not only are these alternatives (particularly surgery) expensive, but also they can pose health risks. By simply making a few changes in your lifestyle, over time you can open the door to weight loss.

YOUR WAISTLINE IS YOUR LIFELINE

I've said it before, but it bears repeating: your waist measurement is more important than your weight. Just as you need to change the way you look at weight loss, you need a different way to look at nutrition. Ask God to help you achieve this outlook. You will be surprised at the way your thinking about food gradually changes. Although I do want you to weigh yourself on a regular basis, I also want you to start looking at your waistline as a key indicator of weight management. This is why the diet I provide in this book is called the Rapid Waist Reduction Diet.

Let's start by reviewing how to measure your waist. Over the years I've discovered that many men do not do this correctly. They may have a 52-inch waist, but they don't realize it because they can still yank on their old jeans with a 32-inch waist. This is only possible because their huge bellies are overlapping their belts while extended use has stretched the fabric beyond normal limits. Yet they insist they have a 32-inch waist.

BMI, Waist Size, and Type 2 Diabetes

Various health organizations, including the Centers for Disease Control and Prevention (CDC) and the National Institutes of Health (NIH), officially define the terms *overweight* and *obesity* using the body mass index (BMI), which factors in a person's weight relative to height. Most of these organizations define an overweight adult as having a BMI between 25 and 29.9, while an obese adult is anyone with a BMI of 30 or higher.[3] If you would like a chart to help you determine your BMI, refer to my book *The Seven Pillars of Health*.

Or do an online search for "BMI" to find tools that can help you calculate yours.

However, an even more important statistic is waist size. The larger your waist, the greater your chances of having type 2 diabetes. For men, waist size is an even better predictor of diabetes than BMI. A thirteen-year study of more than twenty-seven thousand men discovered that:

- A waist size of 34 to 36 inches doubled diabetes risk.

- A waist size of 36 to 38 nearly tripled the risk.

- A waist size of 38 to 40 was associated with five times the risk.

- A waist size of 40 to 62 was associated with twelve times the risk.[4]

In addition, in recent years low-waisted pants became popular in many women's clothing styles. As a result, I have seen more and more women taking their waist measurement way too low.

You should measure your waist around your navel (and love handles, if you have them). Once I showed them where to measure, I have had patients who were shocked by the reality of their true waist measurement. As reality sinks in, I help them devise the following plan to reach their waist measurement goal.

First, establish a waist measurement goal. Initially the waist measurement goal for a man is 40 inches or less. For a woman the goal is 35 inches or less.

Second, take your height in inches and divide it by two. Eventually your waist measurement should be equal to this number or less. In other words, your waist should measure half of your height or less. For example, a 5-foot-10-inch man is 70 inches tall, so his waist around the belly button and love handles should be 35 inches or less.

Notice that this is the *second* step. You need to decrease your waist to 40 inches or less (for men) or 35 inches or less (for women) before you worry about reducing it to half your height.

I realize you are digesting a considerable amount of information in this book (again, pun intended). However, sit down and take things a bite at a time as you formulate your own plans to lose belly fat. The ride may seem all uphill at first, but relax. Over time you will be zipping downhill with the breeze blowing in your face and the frustration of yo-yo diets lost back at the starting line.

Chapter 5

FORGET THE NUMBER
ON THE SCALE

T IM REMEMBERED FITTING into his favorite suit:
the dark blue one his wife had bought for him on
their anniversary trip to Paris. It was the same
one she asked him to wear when they attended a special
banquet or dinner function. A naturally muscular guy
from playing sports during his younger years, Tim had
always had a hard time finding a suit that fit him just
right. Yet this one had. He had to admit that it boosted
his confidence every time he wore it.

Not anymore, though. Now in his midforties, Tim
had not worn this suit for at least eight years. As his
gut expanded, his lean, athletic physique faded into the
annals of history. He had lost most of his confidence, as
I could easily tell when he walked into my office packing
275 pounds on a 5-foot-8-inch frame. Tim had experienced a heart attack the year before and had two coro-
nary artery stents. He suffered from high blood pressure
and excessive cholesterol in his blood, which had forced
him onto numerous medications. It didn't take a doctor
to see he was the picture of poor health.

I told Tim that if he wanted to decrease his chances

of dying early from another heart attack, he needed to lose weight—especially in the abdominal area. His obese, apple-shaped frame held a protruding belly full of toxic fat. Because of it he was at risk for ongoing heart disease, hypertension, type 2 diabetes, metabolic syndrome, and a host of other diseases. Fortunately my warnings motivated him and his wife, and they made a commitment to losing weight. Still Tim admitted to me that he needed a goal, something he could challenge himself with and strive to meet. He also needed new vision, a belief that he could become as thin as the athlete who once darted down the field to victory.

Gastric Banding Surgery

As you set your weight-loss goals, you might be thinking of bariatric surgery—gastric bypass, gastric banding, lap bands—as a weight-loss solution. When a person elects this type of surgery, a silicone band is placed around the upper part of the stomach so that it can only hold about an ounce of food. As a result, the person feels full faster and eats less. The band can be tightened or loosened, depending on an individual's needs. Most people lose about 40 percent of their excess weight with gastric banding; therefore I believe it can be a viable solution. However, it is not the entire solution. Making healthy choices on a daily basis is the only way to maintain weight loss, even when achieved with the help of surgery. If you opt for gastric banding, remember that you must change your eating habits or you may gain the weight back.

Visualizing a New You

The same is true for any person hoping for weight-loss success. In the last chapter I mentioned developing the belief that you can achieve this goal. As part of securing yourself in this new place, try performing a simple mental exercise involving visualization. Picture yourself at a healthy weight. What you consistently visualize and confess, you will eventually become.

Close your eyes, and picture yourself walking around in the body that God intended for you to have—the healthy one. You don't have to shop in plus-size stores any longer. You move easily and confidently and no longer huff and puff when you climb stairs. You will wear a bathing suit with comfort and confidence. Are you catching the vision? It is absolutely essential that you see yourself reaching this healthy weight.

As you visualize yourself weighing a certain weight or being a certain size, you will reset your mental autopilot and start to lose weight. Do not say, "I will lose 30 or 40 pounds by faith," or else you probably will always have 30 or 40 pounds to lose. Instead, say, "I weigh _____" (fill in desired weight).

To boost your efforts, find a photograph of yourself at or near a healthy or desired weight and place it in different areas of your home, such as on the mirror in your bathroom, on your refrigerator, or as a screensaver on your computers at home and in your office. Some people even tape a copy of the picture to their car's steering wheel or dashboard. Regardless of how many places around the house you want to put your healthy or desired weight photo, it is important to put it in a food journal. As you carry your food journal with you throughout the day and look at the picture, visualize yourself becoming that ideal weight again. Confession helps too; each day confess that, by faith, you weigh your desired weight.

SETTING ATTAINABLE GOALS

Success calls for more than verbal proclamations or wishful thinking, though.

When you are about to embark on a significant lifestyle change to lose a significant amount of weight, it is also crucial to establish attainable goals. I have seen countless people launch into a diet with unrealistic goals—and just as many who dive headfirst into a plan with no set goals in mind. Not surprisingly, both wind up failing. Success requires vision, and when it comes to controlling your weight, that vision must incorporate reality.

An unrealistic goal for weight or clothing size sets you up for discouragement. People who get discouraged will usually quit altogether and eventually regain all the weight. For example, if you are a 5-foot-2-inch female and weigh 300 pounds, you are not likely to be a size 2 or 4 a year from now. You may never get that trim. Realistically, look to be a size 10 or 12 with a waist measurement of 35 inches instead of 45. This is an attainable goal. Once you reach it, you can set another.

Likewise, if you hate going to the gym but have set a goal to work out five days a week for an hour per session, you have just created an unrealistic goal and paved the way to failure. Instead, set a goal of ten thousand steps a day on a pedometer, which simply means more movement or walking. Also, avoid making promises that can be easily broken. For instance, do not tell yourself that you will never have another piece of cake, pie, cookie, or whatever food you crave. Whenever you say that, you have set your autopilot on desiring that food and will most likely want it even more. Instead, as you learn how to develop good eating and discipline habits, avoid using the word *never.*

None of this means that you have to settle for lowered expectations. You can and will look better than you ever have. But the important thing is to first set a goal and then keep it in perspective—both of which can come through taking a few initial measurements.

Measuring Up

One of the most important keys to losing weight is establishing attainable goals rather than ones that will leave you frustrated, angry, and most likely *gaining* weight. That's why virtually every physician says that when starting a diet, aim for a goal of losing no more than 10 to 15 percent of your total body weight. Once you've reached that, set a new goal—but don't jump the gun. While you can dream big (or in this case small), remember that traveling on the road to weight loss happens one step at a time.

Baby Steps

To help Tim establish his goals, I weighed him on the scale and then measured his waist, hips, body mass index, and body fat percentage. His BMI was more than 40, his body fat checked in at 32 percent, and his hip measurement came in at only 35 inches. However, these were all secondary to what mattered most at that point for Tim: a waist measurement of 46 inches.

As we started down the road to reducing all these numbers, I shared an important warning: weighing yourself weekly is one of the worst motivators for weight loss. The first few weeks can seem miraculous as individuals watch the pounds fall off and assume this is all "fat-related" weight. The problem is that many people are losing muscle or water weight, which is guaranteed to lower your metabolic rate and eventually sabotage your weight loss. When you reach the inevitable plateau a few weeks or months later and discouragement sets in, you may give up and quit—all because of focusing too much on a daily or weekly scale reading.

I simply had Tim measure his waist, weight, and body fat percentage once a month—while trying on different pants to gauge his shrinking waistline. It didn't take long for him to line up all his old pairs of pants that he had saved, hoping to one day fit into them again. Most important, of course, was getting back into his favorite suit pants he had worn when he weighed almost 100 pounds less and had a 34-inch waist. Because of that, he originally said he wanted to get down to a weight of 185 pounds and a BMI of 28. Although those numbers would have technically kept him in the "overweight" category, I explained to him that because of his naturally muscular frame, even those numbers might cause him to lose muscle and subsequently lower his metabolic rate. Instead, the better way was to establish a goal based on his waist measurement. With this in mind, he set his waist measurement goal at 39 inches, which meant he would lose 7 inches of fat from his abdomen.

Expanding Waists

Over the past four decades, the average American male's waist size has gone from 35 inches to 39 (11 percent). Among women it has increased even more, going from 30 inches to 37 (23 percent). According to the National Institutes of Health, nearly 39 percent of men and 60 percent of women are carrying too much belly fat.[1]

IT'S ALL IN THE WAIST

If you are overweight or obese, I advise you to take the same approach in establishing weight-loss goals. Measure your waistline at your navel or belly button. If you are a man and your waist measurement is 40 inches or more, you are at a much greater risk of heart disease, hypertension, type 2 diabetes, metabolic syndrome, and many other diseases. If you are a woman and your waist measurement is 35 inches or more, you are prone to the same risks. After years of linking only weight and BMI to higher mortality rates and serious illnesses, scientists are understanding—once again—that abdominal fat is a major contributor to the onset of these diseases. Belly fat is highly toxic. After bubble-wrapping itself around internal organs, it secretes powerful inflammatory chemicals that set the stage for type 2 diabetes, heart disease, cancer, and a host of deadly diseases, as well as more weight gain.

Measuring Tools

Although skin calipers are the easiest devices for measuring body fat percentage, they can also be the most inaccurate. For a more precise (albeit it is sometimes expensive) measurement, try:

- Underwater weighing: Fat floats, while lean tissue sinks—making it easy for specialized hydrostatic weighing equipment to get a highly accurate read on how much fat you're actually carrying.

- Dual X-Ray Absorptiometry (DEXA) scan: Using low-level X-rays, this machine takes into consideration your bone mass and muscle mass to calculate your body fat percentage.

- The Bod Pod: A highly accurate (but again expensive) machine that measures how much air you displace.

- Bioelectrical impedance: Less expensive than the other high-tech tools but pricier (and more precise) than a skin caliper, this method measures the speed of an electrical current as it passes through your body. Unfortunately, numerous variables (e.g., full stomach, recent exercise) can sway your results.[2]

That is just one of the reasons your first goal should be to decrease the area holding this toxic fat and keeping you susceptible to disease. After men reduce their waist measurement to 40 inches, their next goal should be to reach 37.5 inches, and eventually their waist measurement goal should be one-half their height in inches or less.

BODY FAT PERCENTAGE

While I see waist size as the most important measurement for establishing weight-loss goals, this does not mean that you can't or shouldn't take other types of measurements—beyond those you can take with a tape measure. Part of the time with patients during their goal-setting stage I spend getting a body fat percentage. I do an initial measurement and then take one a month until they reach their goal.

There are many ways to measure body fat percentage, including a bioimpedance analysis, underwater weighing, and using skinfold calipers. Whatever the method, you need to have your body fat percentage measured the same way each time. Consistency is the key, since the percentage can fluctuate dramatically with inaccurate measurements.

I hold more stock in body fat percentage than I do the body mass index reading. The reason is simple: accuracy. BMI uses only height and weight to judge how overweight or obese a person is. For example, a twenty-three-year-old professional football player and a fifty-six-year-old executive may both be 5 feet 10 inches tall and weigh 220 pounds. This gives both men a BMI of approximately 35, which is considered obese. In reality, however, the player can have a 32-inch waist and a remarkable 6 percent body fat; the executive can have a 44-inch waist and 33 percent body fat. That is an astounding 27 percent differential in body fat percentage alone, which the BMI doesn't take into account.

Hopefully you are beginning to see some of the

confusion that patients, doctors, and other health care workers deal with when it comes to varying measurements. Although many physicians simply use BMI to determine if a person is overweight or obese, I strongly believe more accurate assessments come from using body fat percentage and waist measurements.

Rating your body fat percentage

Finding your ideal body fat percentage involves two main factors: sex and age. According to the American Council on Exercise, a body fat percentage greater than 25 percent in men and greater than 33 percent in women is considered obese. A healthy percent body fat in women is 25–31 percent and in men is 18–25 percent. Initially, obese men should aim for a reading of less than 25 percent, while obese women should shoot for less than 33 percent. Eventually aim for a percent body fat in the healthy range.

However, remember that body fat ranks second to your initial focus to reduce your waist measurement. Don't worry; you will find that body fat percentage will naturally decrease with waist measurement. Also, women should remember—because of their hormones—that they will have a higher body fat percentage than men. Female hormones cause distribution of fat in the breasts, hips, thighs, and buttocks. A typical woman should have between 7 and 10 percent more body fat than the average man. Many health clubs, nutritionists, and physicians have the equipment to measure your percentage of body fat. Once you have this initial number, log it in your food journal and get it checked each month.

However, don't get too hung up on body fat or other measurements like your BMI reading. Focus on one thing and one thing only: waist measurement. Yes, it's that simple. You really do not need a scale or any other fancy tools—just a tape measure. By focusing on your waist and achieving your goal measurement, you will eliminate one of the main risk factors for disease.

A MATTER OF WEIGHT

For some dieters the idea of not looking at a scale every day sounds foreign. Others feel strange if they don't check at least once a week. Yet after helping thousands of individuals lose weight for good, I have seen how most people do better when they either pack up their scale or get rid of it entirely. The reason is almost purely psychological. When dieters lose the wrong type of weight, such as water weight or muscle weight, their skin may sag or wrinkle, their cheeks and eyes may appear hollow, and their muscle mass may melt away. In the meantime, their metabolic rate decreases, their weight plateaus, and they wind up discouraged because each time they hit the scale, the numbers are still the same. Most often these are the people who quit and regain weight.

Five "Non-Digit" Ways to Measure Weight Loss

1. Overall attitude
2. Energy level

3. Fit of clothes

4. Friendly comments and compliments

5. Feeling of taking up less space

Don't get me wrong—weight is important. That is why I always get an initial weight for every patient. Still, because of our weight-obsessed culture, the numbers on a scale can easily become the only measure of success. Though tempting to monitor your progress this way, it is not a reliable indicator of fat loss. And losing fat should be your primary concern. Avoid the potential depression, guilt, shame, or hopelessness by temporarily putting your scale away. Rely more on an old-fashioned tape measure, a pair of old jeans, a food journal, and a monthly body fat percentage measurement while committing to a monthly weigh-in.

Also, weigh yourself on the same day of each month, and make sure you are fully disrobed. If you are a woman, keep in mind that your weight will fluctuate, based on hormonal fluctuations and your menstrual cycle. So do not get discouraged when this occurs.

Once you reach your goal weight, I recommend that you weigh yourself daily. That is the only time that I recommend this, since this is the best way to avoid "slipping."

DAY BY DAY

Now that you have your waist measurement goal and have recorded your body measurements, weight, BMI, and body fat percentage (if desired) in your food journal, you don't have to think about these numbers. Your focus should be on taking things one day at a time. Too many people pay so much attention to the final result that they forget to focus on what they are doing day by day. As a result, they battle discouragement along the way.

If you get nothing else from this chapter, understand that losing weight takes time. Plus, everyone is different and loses weight at different rates. Since they typically have more muscle and a higher metabolic rate, men usually lose much faster than women.

This is one reason to avoid weekly weigh-ins; it is too easy to get discouraged if you only lose a half pound in one week or even gain one because of normal body fluctuations.

Some people gain muscle in the process of losing fat, which often causes their weight loss to go slower. And some individuals are severely metabolically challenged due to chronic dieting, insulin resistance, low thyroid, hormone imbalance, or other factors. This makes each weight-loss experience unique. So don't make the mistake of comparing yourself with someone else who is also trying to lose weight.

You may not be able to control how fast you reach your goal, but you can control how you follow a particular program on a daily basis. When you focus on implementing wise dietary and lifestyle choices day by day, they will eventually become habits. Many experts say that it takes twenty-one days to form a habit. Others think it takes forty; some place it at ninety days. However long it takes, the point is that when you focus on applying principles just for today—without worrying about how you'll face tomorrow or next week—then, over time, it becomes part of your lifestyle. And when that happens, you will find your mind's autopilot set on losing weight. By focusing on one day at a time, you consistently make the right choices. Obviously there will be some exceptional days, such as birthdays, holidays, or anniversaries. You may "cheat" and eat too large a portion of cake or too many high-glycemic foods. Don't let a temporary setback sidetrack you. Remember you are one meal away from getting back on track and again making the right choices.

SUCCESS STORY

The results that Tim saw show that it is possible to set goals and meet them. He achieved his initial waist measurement of 39 inches—a loss of 7 inches—in just six months. Because he had reached that goal, it gave him the momentum and perseverance to establish another goal. This is often the case with obese people who are able to lose weight, which is why I emphasize setting realistic, attainable goals. Tim's second goal was getting to a waist measurement of 35 inches, which he attained in just four months.

Tim's weight decreased from 275 pounds to 210 pounds in less than a year. (And imagine how good that felt.) More importantly, he lost 11 inches of waist girth during that time, and his blood sugar levels returned to normal. And his blood pressure and cholesterol also normalized without any medication. He was more active and had more energy at any time since he was young. He combined laserlike vision with realistic goals. In the process he avoided serious health issues that were sure to follow had he continued down the path of obesity.

Chapter 6

PREPARING FOR THE RAPID WAIST REDUCTION DIET

S TILL WONDERING IF this book will deliver on the promise to decrease your waist measurement? With the program I now call my Rapid Waist Reduction Diet (RWRD), I have helped countless patients over the years to lose weight. I've seen this program work for them, and I know it can work for you too.

I'm going to outline the program for you in chapters 7 and 8, but first I want you to understand how I came to develop a weight-loss program that can deliver such an amazing promise and also share important information you need to know before proceeding further and embarking on the program.

HOW THE RWRD PROGRAM WAS DEVELOPED

It all actually began over sixty years ago when Dr. A. T. W. Simeons developed a low-calorie diet and worked on his protocol for approximately twenty years. His protocol, *Pounds and Inches*, was published in 1954. He discovered that when his 500-calorie-a-day, very low-fat and very low-carbohydrate diet was combined with small daily doses of the pregnancy hormone hCG (human chorionic gonadotropin), it caused the body to release abnormal collections of fat in the problem areas of the hips, thighs, buttocks, waist, and belly.

In Dr. Simeons's day patients were hospitalized for in-patient treatment for the entire six-week duration of the program. Many consider Dr. Simeons's protocol the best-kept medical secret as well as the most effective weight-loss program of all time.

Typically patients on the protocol report having high energy levels, a sense of well-being, and little to no hunger. According to Dr. Simeons, 60 to 70 percent of the patients kept the weight off long-term.

In 2007 consumer advocate Kevin Trudeau made Dr. Simeons's protocol known to the world in his book *The Weight Loss Cure "They" Don't Want You to Know About*. I started recommending the Simeons Protocol and monitoring patients back in 2008. At that time I used hCG injections. However, now I recommend either the sublingual hCG tab that is compounded by a compounding pharmacy or homeopathic hCG drops.* (The homeopathic hCG drops may be difficult to find due to new regulations, but they are available.) The Food and Drug Administration (FDA) requires us to inform patients of the following statement: "hCG has not been

---

* As of the printing of this book, the FDA does not allow over-the-counter (OTC) hCG drops to be labeled as homeopathic and make claims about weight loss. It is extremely difficult to get homeopathic hCG drops due to the new FDA regulations The drops I recommend have been modified to comply with the FDA. The prescription sublingual hCG tabs I recommend also comply with the FDA restrictions as they are prescribed and not OTC and this new regulation does not pertain to the prescription sublingual hCG drops.

demonstrated to be an effective adjunctive therapy in the treatment of obesity. There is no substantial evidence that it increases weight loss beyond that resulting from calorie restriction, that it causes a more attractive or 'normal' distribution of fat or that it decreases the hunger and discomfort associated with calorie restricted diets." For women who are still menstruating, I recommend that they start the hCG sublingual tablets when their menstrual period stops; if they are on the protocol for six weeks, they need to go off of the hCG sublingual tablets during their menstrual period.

The first two days of the protocol you need to take the hCG and eat as many good fats and calories as possible, such as salads with lots of organic extra-virgin olive oil, organic peanut butter, almond butter, avocadoes, hummus, guacamole, seeds, nuts, coconut oil, and other healthy fats. During these two days eat as much fat as you can every three hours.

Results do vary from person to person, but a number of my patients have been able to come off all their medications after following the RWRD and losing belly fat. I have modified the 500 calories in the Simeons Protocol to approximately 1,000 calories in the RWRD, but I've kept Simeons's ratio of proteins, fats, and carbohydrates the same. I have also added more soluble fiber and supplements to boost serotonin levels since low-carbohydrate diets are usually associated with low serotonin levels. Adding soluble fiber also helps with satiety, blood sugar control, and improved bowel movements. This program has been very effective for my patients, and I call it phase one of my Rapid Waist Reduction

Diet, which I will outline in chapter 7. Phase one typically lasts four to six weeks and is followed by phase two, which I have outlined in chapter 8. Dr. Simeons also allowed very small amounts of wheat in his diet (such as Melba toast and Grissini breadsticks), so I have allowed them as well. However, when you are on the anti-inflammatory diet, I remove all wheat products.

Make Sure You Can Participate

Certain people cannot participate in the RWRD. Please read the following very carefully and be sure to get the permission of your primary care physician before attempting to follow this protocol. You must be eighteen years of age or older, and certain medical conditions, medications, and supplements may exclude you as a candidate.

Medical Conditions That May Exclude You From This Program

- Pregnant or planning to become pregnant
- Currently breastfeeding
- Surgery—you must be off the RWRD a minimum of two weeks before having surgery. If you have recently had surgery, you must wait a full six weeks before starting the RWRD, and you must inform your surgeon about being on the program prior to surgery.
- Cancer of any kind, except for certain skin cancers
- Heart failure

- Type 1 diabetes—however, people with type 2 diabetes can participate with the consent of a physician since this protocol can possibly reverse their medical condition.

- Chronic renal failure

- Severe anemia

- Epilepsy or any other seizure disorders

- Mental illness, including moderate to severe depression; moderate to severe anxiety; suicidal thoughts, ideations, or attempts; bipolar disorder; or psychosis

---

Medications That May Exclude You From This Program

- Diuretics

- Anti-inflammatory medications

- Coumadin

- Insulin

- Birth control—birth control pills will not work with this program.

All other prescription medications, over-the-counter medications, and nutritional supplements must be cleared by your medical doctor prior to starting the RWRD.

I also want to remind you that if you are prediabetic or diabetic, you must talk to your personal health care practitioner before making any changes to your diet, natural supplements, or medications. The advice in this book is based on general principles of health, but your physician knows your individual situation and needs to be involved to ensure the steps you take to incorporate these principles into your dietary program are done in a way that will work for your particular health needs.

Also, while this is a temporary protocol to help you lose belly fat, it is only the first step in a lifestyle change. The goal of having more than one phase of the diet is to help you stabilize your weight and then return to normal meals that follow healthy eating guidelines. If you are going to maintain your weight loss, you will have to stick with a healthy way of eating for the long haul. It is the key to keeping obesity and disease at bay and enabling you to live the healthy, abundant life you were designed to live.

In my opinion, by creating two phases of this program, I have combined the best weight-loss program with the best maintenance program. Again, results vary, but according to Dr. Simeons, patients who strictly adhere to his protocol typically experience a 1-pound-per-day loss of weight. Since I have doubled the calorie content, one will typically lose approximately half of a pound a day. According to Dr. Simeons, his protocol allows your body to maintain its structural fat, which helps prevent sagging skin and a drawn, tired-looking face. The skin may actually glow and may appear more youthful.

THE DIET TO END ALL DIETS

I'm not a proponent of dieting. However, because patients I've treated with the RWRD program typically experience consistent, steady weight loss, which keeps them very motivated while they practice incorporating the key dietary and lifestyle components they'll need to maintain their weight loss, I feel this diet puts an end to all other dieting. My goal is to get you committed to a healthy lifestyle program that will give you the best quality of life possible, and I believe the two phases of this program will result in you no longer being caught in the vicious cycle of yo-yo dieting. I believe the Rapid Waist Reduction Diet is the last diet you will ever need.

As the name reflects, the focus of this program is reducing your waist measurement. Although I have reviewed such topics as calories, fat grams, and glycemic index values, you *won't* track any of these things during phase one or phase two. Instead, during phase one you will learn to select the right type and amount of low-glycemic carbohydrates and combine them with the right amounts of healthy proteins while avoiding most fats. This combination will literally program your body to burn fat, particularly the toxic fat in your belly. During phase two healthy anti-inflammatory fats will be added in the correct proportions to healthy low-glycemic carbohydrates and healthy proteins.

There are some risks you need to be aware of before you begin.

Understanding the Risks

In my practice I have patients read the following risks before signing a consent form to begin this program. I believe this information is important for you to know before you agree to participate in the Rapid Waist Reduction Diet.

- I understand the side effects of hCG administration and a low-calorie/nonfat diet can include dizziness, light-headedness, and lowered blood pressure.

- I understand that my blood pressure must be checked at least two times a week.

- I understand that I must be under the care of my primary care physician during the entire cycle of hCG supplementation (four to six weeks).

- I understand that taking diuretics, anti-inflammatory drugs, or Coumadin will require monitoring blood tests, as determined by my physician.

- I understand that there is a limit of 1,000 calories allowed daily on this diet.

- I understand that increasing my caloric intake could alter the results and increase medical risks.

- I understand that cheating by eating sugary or fatty foods while on phase one can be harmful and may predispose me to forming gallstones.

- I consent to taking sublingual hCG. I agree to be monitored by medical professionals during my weight-loss treatment period. My primary care provider will also monitor any medical condition not related to the RWRD.

- I understand that the FDA has *not* approved hCG for weight loss and that there is no medical data that support the use of hCG for weight-loss purposes.

- I understand that I will be required to have current (within one month of beginning the RWRD program) lab test results on my chart. These tests are performed to rule out any conditions that could be worsened by the stringent caloric restriction and/or the administration of sublingual hCG in the RWRD program.

- I agree to report any problems or side effects that occur within the time frame of treatment to my medical professionals.

- I understand that I must have an established relationship with a primary care provider before starting this program

- I understand that I must consult with my primary care provider to receive refills on medications that were prescribed by them. Doing so will help minimize confusion between patients and medical providers.

- I understand that the following conditions may prohibit intake of a low-calorie diet:

  - History of recent myocardial infarction (MI)/heart attack

  - History of CVAs (stroke) and/or TIAs

  - Uncontrolled seizures

  - Unstable angina, clotting disorders, or DVT/PE

  - Severe diabetes

  - Severe liver disease (may require a low-protein diet)

  - Severe kidney disease (may require a low-protein diet)

  - Active peptic ulcer disease

  - Active cancers

- • Pregnancy, actively trying to become pregnant, or currently breast feeding

- • Eating disorder (e.g., anorexia nervosa or bulimia)

- • Severe psychiatric disturbance (e.g., major depression and/or suicide attempts, bipolar disorder, or psychosis)

- • Corticosteroid therapy greater than 20 milligrams a day

- • Chronic illicit drug usage, addictions, alcoholism, substance abuse

- • I understand that failure to comply with protocols—including keeping my primary care physician advised of my medical history, this regimen, and any changes in my condition—may predispose me to develop gallbladder disease, sabotage my weight-loss goals, or cause other harm.

Benefits of Detoxing Before the RWRD

I typically have patients detox for a month prior to phase one to enhance the success of the RWRD program. I believe that preparing your body for the very low-calorie diet and hCG phase of the program is an absolute must.

Your body can harbor a host of unpleasant substances, including, but not limited to, pesticides, herbicides, parasites, candida, and heavy metals. Toxins usually are stored in the dense fat that will be released during phase one of the RWRD program. If all the toxins from the liver, colon, and fat were released at once, the results could be detrimental to your health.

In addition, most overweight people are actually nutritionally deficient. I have found that ridding the body of toxins, parasites, yeast, and fungus, in addition to restoring it nutritionally, ensures success of the RWRD program. I believe an entire month (thirty days) is needed in order to get your body ready for phase one, so I highly recommend you participate in a thirty-day detox program before beginning the RWRD program. The thirty-day detox diet is simply my anti-inflammatory diet or candida diet and eating only organic foods. Refer to *The Bible Cure for Candida and Yeast Infections* for more information, or read chapters 2 and 3 again in this book.

Results vary from one individual to the next, but my patients who have gone through thirty days of detoxification before starting the RWRD program usually report the following benefits:

- Improved mental clarity
- Flatter abdomen
- Decreased appetite and cravings
- Improved mood
- Improved energy level
- Feeling of overall vitality and better health

- Weight loss of between 5 and 30 pounds while detoxing

- Acceleration of the rate of weight loss in RWRD phase one

I have carefully determined that taking the following supplements for a month prior to phase one will help detox your body, rid it of parasites and candida, and boost your nutritional status. For information on where to order these products, see Appendix B.

- Beta TCP: Two tablets three times a day. This will help support gallbladder function, which usually becomes sluggish with age.

- Divine Health Living Multivitamin: One scoop in the morning. This supplement is loaded with vitamins, minerals, antioxidants, and phytonutrients. Or you can take Max N-Fuse.

- Divine Health Probiotic: Two capsules in the morning on an empty stomach. This restores beneficial, healthy bacteria to your gastrointestinal tract.

- Divine Health Fiber Formula: One heaping teaspoon in 4 ounces of water every night at bedtime. This assists in cleansing the intestines of toxins, and it also aids in regularity of bowel movements.

- Vitamin D$_3$: 2,000 IUs a day assists the immune system.

- Living Omega: One capsule two times a day. This is pharmaceutical-grade fish oil that supports cardiovascular, brain, joint, and eye health.

- Cellgevity: Two capsules two times a day. This supports liver detoxification and has antioxidant and anti-inflammatory protection.

While on this month-long detox program, I encourage you to eat only organic food if possible to prevent recontamination of toxins in your body. Weight training and brisk aerobic exercise are highly recommended during this thirty-day detox as well, but only mild walking is recommended during phase one of the RWRD. Once you have successfully completed thirty days of detoxing, you are ready for phase one, which is based on a modification of the Simeons Protocol.

Chapter 7

RAPID WAIST REDUCTION DIET, PHASE ONE

B EFORE STARTING PHASE one of the Rapid Waist Reduction Diet, take your photo and record your weight, blood pressure, and BMI. Make certain your primary care physician monitors your blood pressure if you are taking medication for hypertension. *Your blood pressure usually lowers significantly during treatment.* Here are a few other suggestions you should follow:

- Only take medications (including over-the-counter medications) specified by your primary care physician, who should monitor and adjust dosing as needed.

- Supplements can help with overall health during the protocol, including PGX fiber, Divine Health Fiber Formula, Serotonin Max, Divine Health Living Multivitamin or Max N-Fuse, and Cellgevity. (See Appendix B.)

- Strictly follow the following list of approved foods. Phase one of the Rapid Waist Reduction Diet is a 1,000-calorie-a-day diet that starts on the third day you begin taking hCG, sublingual tab or homeopathic drops. It needs to be followed exactly.

- Do *not* attempt this diet without the hCG. The slightest variation can prevent weight loss. If you find that the hCG drops are not enough to curb your appetite, it is fine to take both drops and sublingual tabs at the same time. This should be very effective in controlling your appetite as you stick to the eating plan.

PHASE ONE EATING GUIDELINES

Dr. Simeons would place his patients on a 500-calorie-a-day diet with injections of hCG and would hospitalize his patients for the entire six-week duration of the program. I have found over the years that the majority of my patients would not stay on the 500-calorie-a-day diet, nor would they fulfill their commitment to twice-a-week checkups at my office. I then decided to modify his program for my patients and simply doubled the calorie intake to 1,000 calories a day. Since most of my patients either skipped breakfast or ate a light breakfast, I added a choice for breakfast of either a meal consisting of meat and vegetables or fruit or a specific type of protein drink.

There are many different foods, especially fruits and vegetables, that have the same calories or even lower calories than the fruits and vegetables listed; however, they interfere with weight loss on the hCG program. This is why it's important that you commit to eating only approved foods. Here are some helpful tips to keep in mind:

- When choosing meats, always choose the leanest cuts of organic meats and trim off all of the fat.

- All of your foods and beverages need to be organic.

- Tea, coffee, and clean pure water and mineral water are the only drinks allowed.

- Drink coffee or tea in any amount (no sugar and only 1 tablespoon of skim milk is allowed every twenty-four hours). To sweeten, stevia is preferred, but saccharin is allowed.

- You should drink at least 2 quarts of water daily. However, you can drink more than that. Good waters include spring water (such as Mountain Valley Spring Water). Your body may retain water when your water intake falls below its normal requirements. This in turn may slow down your weight loss.

- If you feel dizzy or light-headed during this diet, increase your intake of water, and take PGX fiber with each meal.

- The fruit or the melba toast may be eaten between meals instead of with lunch or dinner, but no more than four items listed for lunch and dinner may be eaten at one meal. Take PGX fiber, two capsules with 8–16 ounces of water if you eat the fruit or melba toast between meals.

- You may have a Grissini breadstick and an apple for breakfast or an orange before bedtime, but these must be deducted from your lunch or dinner rations. (Dr. Simeons preferred the Italian breadsticks called Grissini, which are more satisfying than melba toast.)

- Do not eat your daily ration of two breads and two fruits at the same time. Ingesting too many carbohydrates at one time slows down weight loss. You may not save food from one day to eat the next.

- There is no restriction on the size of one apple.

- Variants for the meat protein: You may occasionally eat 100 grams or 3½ ounces of fat-free cottage cheese. (No other cheese is allowed.) You may occasionally

eat one whole egg with three egg whites
in place of a meat portion.

• All fat must be trimmed from the raw
meat before weighing. Only meats listed
are permitted.

• If it is not on the list, *do not eat it in any
quantity*. Dr. Simeons spent many years
developing this program and found that
even substituting okra, artichokes, and so
on, although of equivalent caloric value,
did not produce equivalent results. There
is no need to reinvent the wheel. There
will be plenty of time for creativity when
you get to phase two.

• All meat must be broiled or boiled.

• Vegetables must be raw or steamed.

• The juice of one lemon is allowed for all
purposes.

• A small amount of salt, pepper, vinegar, mustard powder, garlic, sweet basil,
parsley, thyme, marjoram, and so forth
may be used as desired for seasoning, but
no oil, butter, or dressing.

• All fresh white fish must be low in mercury (catfish, cod, haddock, herring,
mullet, sardine, tilapia, tongol tuna,
whitefish, whiting).

- A George Foreman grill and steamer would be very helpful.

OTHER CONSIDERATIONS

- *No creams, oils, or lotions* should be used on your face, skin, or body during this program. Topically applied hormones should be in gel form (no creams or oils).

- *No cosmetics* other than lipstick, eyebrow pencil, mascara, and powder should be used. During this time you should use one of the many all-mineral powder cosmetics, such as Bare Minerals, for your foundation.

- *No massages:* The use of a far-infrared sauna is encouraged instead.

- *Sunshine:* Try to get at least five to ten minutes of sun every day.

- *Female cycles:* If you are a menstruating female, you cannot use the hCG sublingual tablets during your menstrual period. I have patients stop taking hCG sublingual tablets during their menstrual period; however, patients usually do not need to do this with the homeopathic drops.

- *Pedometer:* Make sure you get mild exercise in every day. Wearing a pedometer

will help to ensure you get your ten thousand steps in for the day.

• *Constipation:* If you experience constipation during the diet, use Divine Health
Fiber Formula, 1 heaping teaspoon a day
with water. (See Appendix B.)

REPEATING CYCLES IF YOU HAVE MORE WEIGHT TO LOSE

Cycle one: First round of hCG

• If you have a small amount of belly fat to
lose, then do phase one for four weeks.
As soon as the toxic belly fat is gone, you
will usually begin to feel hungry again.
After losing the toxic fat, you need to go
to the phase two program.

• If you have more belly fat to lose, then
you can follow phase one for about six
weeks.

• If you stop losing weight during phase
one, then switch the diet to six Granny
Smith apples (no other foods) per day with
plenty of water. When you begin losing
weight again, resume the phase one diet.

Cycle two: Another round of hCG, if needed

- If you need another cycle of hCG, then you should begin again after six weeks of being on the phase two program.

Repeated cycles of hCG:

- If you need to repeat several cycles of hCG because you still have weight to lose, you need to wait eight weeks before cycle three. If you have more to lose, wait twelve weeks before cycle four. If you need another cycle, wait twenty weeks before cycle five, and wait six months before cycle six.

APPROVED FOODS FOR PHASE ONE

Start the following diet and continue it for the next four to six weeks, depending on the amount of weight you need to lose. Choose only from the following approved foods for each meal. You should choose different foods for each meal and from day to day. A seven-day meal plan follows this list of approved foods. The meal plan is an example you can use to plan out what you will eat a week at a time.

For breakfast you may substitute a protein shake that contains 18 to 25 grams of protein, less than 3 grams of sugar, and less than 2 grams of fat. (See Appendix B.) You may blend the protein with 8 ounces of water, 8 ounces of unsweetened almond milk (found at most health food stores), 4 ounces of So Delicious unsweetened, nonfat coconut milk with 4 ounces of water, or 8 ounces of water with 1 tablespoon of skim milk. You may also blend ½ cup of frozen strawberries. Another breakfast option, only one time a week, is one egg (omega-3 or pasteurized) with two additional egg whites cooked with a small amount of Pam cooking spray or poached (which is preferred). You may accompany the egg and egg whites with melba toast and fruit.

NOTE: You should choose a different meat and vegetable for lunch and dinner on the same day. You may choose to eat your fruit as a midafternoon snack.

APPROVED FOODS FOR PHASE ONE	
Beverages	• Water • Tea • Coffee (See guidelines for allowable sweetener and milk.)
Lean Meat/ Protein (grilled or boiled, 3.5 oz., or 100 g; choose one per meal)	• Lobster • Veal • Beef • Chicken breast • Crab • Fresh white fish • Shrimp • Bison (buffalo) • Elk • Venison (deer) • Egg (you may occasionally have an egg, either hardboiled or scrambled with a small amount of cooking spray with two additional egg whites)

APPROVED FOODS FOR PHASE ONE	
Vegetables (raw or steamed, 1 cup; choose one per meal)	• Spinach • Chard • Chicory • Beet greens • Green salad • Tomato • Celery • Fennel • Onions • Red radishes • Cucumbers • Asparagus • Cabbage
Fruits (choose one per meal)	• Apple • Granny Smith apple • ½ grapefruit • ½ cup strawberries (You may choose to eat your fruit for a meal or for a snack.)
Breads	• 2 Grissini breadsticks (see Appendix B) • 2 slices melba toast

Seven-Day Meal Plan for Phase One

Remember, the first two days of the phase one protocol you need to take the hCG and eat as many good fats and calories as possible, such as salads with lots of organic extra-virgin olive oil, organic peanut butter, almond butter, avocadoes, hummus, guacamole, seeds, nuts, coconut oil, and other healthy fats. During these two days eat as much fat as you can every three hours. What follows is a seven-day meal plan that begins on day 3.

Day 3

Breakfast

- Fresh white fish (3.5 oz. for women or 6 oz. for men) OR one egg, hard boiled or poached. You can make an omelet using Pam cooking spray, adding onions, tomato, spinach, chicory, and celery, with salt and pepper to taste. Do NOT include cheese or mushrooms.
- 1 apple
- OR protein shake with fruit

Lunch

- Chicken breast (3.5 oz. for women or 6 oz. for men)
- 1 cup spinach or green salad
- 2 Grissini breadsticks or 2 slices melba toast
- ½ cup strawberries or ½ grapefruit

Dinner

- Lean beef, elk, buffalo, veal, or filet mignon (3.5 oz. for women or 6 oz. for men)
- 1 cup green salad or asparagus
- 2 Grissini breadsticks or 2 slices melba toast

Day 4

Breakfast

- 1 egg and 2 extra egg whites
- ½ grapefruit
- OR protein shake with fruit

Lunch

- Fresh white fish (3.5 oz. for women or 6 oz. for men)
- 1 cup cabbage or green salad
- 2 Grissini breadsticks or 2 slices melba toast
- ½ cup strawberries

Dinner

- Crab or shrimp (3.5 oz. for women or 6 oz. for men)
- 1 cup asparagus or green salad
- 2 Grissini breadsticks or 2 slices melba toast

Day 5

Breakfast

- Fresh white fish (3.5 oz. for women or 6 oz. for men) OR one egg, hard boiled or poached. You can make an omelet using Pam cooking spray, adding onions, tomato, spinach, chicory, and celery, with salt and pepper to taste. Do NOT include cheese or mushrooms.
- 1 Granny Smith apple
- OR protein shake with fruit

Lunch

- Chicken breast (3.5 oz. for women or 6 oz. for men)
- 1 cup tomatoes or green salad
- 2 Grissini breadsticks or 2 slices melba toast
- ½ cup strawberries

Dinner

- Deer, elk, veal, or filet mignon (3.5 oz. for women or 6 oz. for men)
- 1 cup spinach or green salad
- 2 Grissini breadsticks or 2 slices melba toast

Day 6

Breakfast

- Fresh white fish (3.5 oz. for women or 6 oz. for men) OR one egg, hard boiled or poached. You can make an omelet using Pam cooking spray, adding onions, tomato, spinach, chicory, and celery, with salt and pepper to taste. Do NOT include cheese or mushrooms.
- ½ grapefruit
- OR protein shake with fruit

Lunch

- Chicken breast (3.5 oz. for women or 6 oz. for men)
- 1 cup romaine salad with up to 5 sprays of Wishbone salad spritzer
- 2 Grissini breadsticks or 2 slices melba toast
- ½ cup strawberries

Dinner

- Filet mignon (3.5 oz. for women or 6 oz. for men)
- 1 cup spinach or green salad
- 2 Grissini breadsticks or 2 slices melba toast

Day 7

Breakfast

- Shrimp (3.5 oz. for women or 6 oz. for men) OR one egg, hard boiled or poached. You can make an omelet using Pam cooking spray, adding onions, tomato, spinach, chicory, and celery, with salt and pepper to taste. Do NOT include cheese or mushrooms.
- 1 apple
- OR protein shake with fruit

Lunch

- Fresh white fish (3.5 oz. for women or 6 oz. for men)
- 1 cup cucumbers or green salad
- 2 Grissini breadsticks or 2 slices melba toast
- ½ grapefruit

Dinner

- Veal, filet mignon, or extra lean hamburger meat (3.5 oz. for women or 6 oz. for men)
- 1 cup mixed greens salad or asparagus
- 2 Grissini breadsticks or 2 slices melba toast

Day 8

Breakfast

- Fresh white fish (3.5 oz. for women or 6 oz. for men) OR one egg, hard boiled or poached. You can make an omelet using Pam cooking spray, adding onions, tomato, spinach, chicory, and celery, with salt and pepper to taste. Do NOT include cheese or mushrooms.

- ½ cup strawberries
- OR protein shake with fruit

Lunch

- Chicken breast (3.5 oz. for women or 6 oz. for men)
- 1 cup green salad
- 2 Grissini breadsticks or 2 slices melba toast
- ½ grapefruit

Dinner

- Crab (3.5 oz. for women or 6 oz. for men)
- 1 cup spinach
- 2 Grissini breadsticks or 2 slices melba toast

Day 9

Breakfast

- 1 hardboiled egg
- ½ cup strawberries

Lunch

- Chicken breast (3.5 oz. for women or 6 oz. for men)
- 1 cup green salad
- 2 Grissini breadsticks or 2 slices melba toast
- 1 Granny Smith apple

Dinner

- Lean beef (3.5 oz. for women or 6 oz. for men)
- 1 cup red radishes or salad
- 2 Grissini breadsticks or 2 slices melba toast

Chapter 8

RAPID WAIST REDUCTION DIET, PHASE TWO

CONGRATULATIONS! YOU HAVE completed the toughest phase. Now is the time for you to get creative with your food choices. You may eat any free-range and organic foods you like except for sugars and starches. Starches include potatoes, corn, grains (including breads and pasta), or any food including these choices. Sugars include honey, molasses, maple syrup, corn syrup, and, of course, sugar.

You will be on this phase for at least six weeks. At the end of these six weeks, if you have more belly fat to lose, then you will need to repeat another hCG cycle (phase one). However, if you have lost most of your belly fat and your blood sugars are normal, you can begin simply following the principles of the anti-inflammatory diet I outlined in chapters 2 and 3.

Once you move on to the anti-inflammatory diet, make sure you weigh yourself daily. If your weight starts to climb, you will need to repeat this six-week phase two program. If belly fat starts collecting, then you will need to go back on phase one.

I've divided phase two in to two sub-phases. Why?

It takes three weeks for your new, lower weight to stabilize. It would be a shame to ruin your hard work by reintroducing sugars and starches too quickly.

Therefore phase two has a no carbohydrate stage for three weeks. Beginning with week four, a few healthy carbohydrates such as beans, peas, lentils, oatmeal, and high-fiber cereals are allowed. You can begin using unsweetened almond milk or unsweetened nonfat coconut milk (instead of cow's milk). You don't *have* to add these starches back into your diet in week four; you might find you no longer desire them, which is perfectly fine.

Once a healthy waist size is reached and blood sugars are controlled, you can then follow an anti-inflammatory diet, but you will always need to avoid sugar and desserts. You will also need to weigh yourself daily and go back on phase one or two if you start gaining weight again.

What to Do if You Aren't Losing Weight

If for some reason you are not achieving optimal results with the RWRD program, you may need one of the following tests. Talk to your primary care physician or refer to Appendix B for information on these tests.

- NeuroScience Adrenal to test your neurotransmitters and adrenal function
- Hormone testing
- ALCAT food sensitivity testing
- Anxiety/depression testing

- Thyroid hormone testing
- Further metabolic testing
- Yeast/candida testing

EATING GUIDELINES FOR PHASE TWO

Breakfast

I can't overemphasize that breakfast is the most important meal of the day and a key to weight loss. I have already mentioned the importance of fiber and its role in controlling appetite. Getting enough fiber at breakfast is also instrumental to stabilizing your blood sugar for hours, boosting energy, and keeping your mind sharp and digestive system working optimally. I often call fiber nature's street sweeper for your GI tract.

To control hunger and keep your GI tract functioning optimally during phase two, you should eat 5 to 10 grams of fiber per meal and 3 to 6 grams in a snack, with a mixture of soluble and insoluble fiber. Since most people consume so little fiber, let me also offer a word of caution. Starting with 10 grams of fiber a meal may cause excessive gas and abdominal discomfort. Don't worry—your body will adjust. However, you may need to gradually increase intake by starting with 5 grams and possibly working up to 10. I use fiber supplements with meals and snacks to insure that one is getting adequate fiber, and by taking a fiber supplement before meals, it many times helps control appetite. After avoiding starches for the first three weeks of phase two, you can begin eating unsweetened steel-cut oatmeal with stevia, Just Like Sugar, or xylitol, which are natural sweeteners.

Lunch and dinner

I've grouped lunch and dinner together because I want to promote a different mind-set, one that grasps that these meals are secondary to breakfast. Although there may be a wider variety of items to choose from for lunch and dinner than there are at breakfast, that is simply because most of our "taste buds" are a little more expansive later in the day. We don't typically wake up craving apples, asparagus, or sweet potatoes. Don't confuse having more options with thinking you need to eat more at these meals.

Carbs

Remember: no carbs such as pasta, rice, bread, or starchy vegetables for the first three weeks of phase two. This period is carbohydrate free. Starting with week four, you may have beans, peas, and legumes with your meals. However, for all six weeks of phase two you can have as many non-starchy vegetables as desired. You may also sprinkle Butter Buds or Molly McButter on them, or use Smart Balance Butter Burst spray to improve the taste and flavor of your vegetables. Or you can season them with spices.

Proteins

Generally most meats and fish contain approximately 7 grams of protein per ounce. I recommend 2 to 6 ounces of protein per serving—2 to 4 for women and 3 to 6 for men, depending on lean body mass and activity level.

Some species of fish contain more mercury, PCBs (polychlorinated biphenyls), and other contaminants. Fish that are higher in mercury include shark, swordfish, king mackerel, and tilefish. Albacore tuna and canned tuna contain moderate amounts. Fish low in mercury include haddock, herring, Atlantic mackerel, ocean perch, pollack, salmon (both fresh and canned), sardines, tilapia, trout, and tongol tuna.

Young children, pregnant women, women who may become pregnant, or women who are nursing should avoid eating fish high in mercury. The American College of Obstetricians and Gynecologists recommends a maximum of two 6-ounce servings of fish each week for pregnant women.[1] The American Academy of Pediatrics recommends children and nursing women consume no more than 7 ounces of high-mercury-level fish per week.[2] Realize that all fish increasingly contain more mercury, which is toxic to fetuses and to children's brains. In addition, farm-raised fish are generally prone to containing more PCBs than wild fish.

Fats

It is best to choose salad spritzers that are very, very low in fat. During the rapid waist reduction phase we must restrict fat to the bare minimum in order to burn belly fat as well as grains and most other complex carbohydrates. I also recommend the new low-fat salad spritzers sold in supermarkets, including Wishbone and Ken's Lite Accents brands. They have only one calorie per spray; in my opinion they are superior to other salad dressing options. Nonfat dressings are an option, but most people do not enjoy their taste—and enjoying what you eat is crucial to your success. Most patients enjoy one of the new salad spritzers with only 1 calorie per spray.

Making a Meal

As an example, let's construct either a lunch or dinner using some of the items just listed. To start with a beverage, you can drink a glass of spring water, filtered water, or sparkling water with a squeeze of lemon or lime. You may also drink tea sweetened with stevia or Just Like Sugar and a squeeze of lemon or lime.

Keep salads healthy

When eating out, skip the bread and start your meal with a salad made of large, dark-green leaves and plenty of cucumbers, tomatoes, raw carrots, and onions. You may add brussels sprouts or broccoli spears. Then add ten or more sprays of a salad spritzer. I believe the easiest way to cut fat is to use a salad spritzer with only minimal fat per spray. Be careful to stick to salad spritzers since this minimizes your fat intake. Leave off the cheese and croutons.

Most people forget that 10 cups of romaine lettuce has only about 100 calories, while a mere 1-½ tablespoons of most salad dressings contain an equivalent amount of calories. People hoping to lose weight often get into trouble by eating salads smothered with high-calorie salad dressings. A large Caesar salad may only have 10 calories in the salad leaves but more than 1,000 calories worth of dressing.

Soup is not an option

Next up for your meal is a soup. Select a low-sodium, broth-based kind, such as vegetable or bean. These are very filling and will usually prevent you from over-eating. Avoid cream-based soups, such as clam chowder or broccoli cheddar, which are high in calories. Make sure your soup is low in sodium (preferably less than 500 milligrams) and low in fat (less than 10 grams). One of the key ingredients for a healthy soup is fiber, so look for those that have at least 3 grams. When it comes to fiber, the higher the better. Finally, don't overdo it on the carbohydrate content. Many soups are loaded with high-glycemic carbs, such as white rice and pasta. Choose vegetable soups, such as minestrone or black bean. Make sure for dinner you choose only vegetable soups.

If, by chance, you are still extremely hungry after salad and soup, you can take some fiber capsules. Take two to four PGX fiber capsules—again with 16 ounces of water. When you do this before you eat your entree, you fill your stomach faster and are less likely to overeat the wrong types of foods.

Guidelines for entrees

Stick with the guidelines mentioned previously of a 2- to 4-ounce serving of protein for women and 3 to 8 ounces for men. For example, try a grilled chicken breast flavored with low-sodium seasonings. (Watch out for high-carb, high-calorie marinades.) Along with your main source of protein, add a serving of vegetables, such as broccoli, which should take up about half of your plate.

Next, select a low-glycemic starch, such as ½ cup for women and 1 cup for men of beans, peas, lentils, legumes, or sweet potatoes. While women can have one serving and men one and a half to two servings of starch for breakfast and lunch, they should avoid starch and fruit for dinner except for beans, peas, and lentils. In addition, you can end your meal (except dinner) with a piece of low-glycemic fruit.

If you are eating out, remember that most entree serving sizes are double or triple the recommended serving size. Simply eat half the protein and low-glycemic starch, and save the rest for another meal or snack. Or ask if you can share with another person at the table.

Save desserts for special occasions

After reaching your goal waist measurement, on very rare occasions you may eat a treat, i.e., dark chocolate or another very small dessert. Prior to enjoying a dessert, I recommend that you take two to four PGX fiber capsules with 16 ounces of water. This not only lowers the dessert's glycemic index value, but it also helps you feel fuller. With desserts it is especially important to practice mindfulness and savor each bite so that you do not overeat and sabotage weight-loss efforts. If you do eat dessert, it's best to eat it for lunch or at an early dinner (before four o'clock) and decrease your starch intake for that meal. Also, take PGX fiber afterward.

APPROVED FOODS FOR PHASE TWO

Low-glycemic, non-grain carbs (three to four servings per day—breakfast, lunch, and snacks; no carbs after 6:00 p.m. except non-starchy vegetables or "green carbs," which are unlimited)	
Legumes and Beans and Starches Serving = ½ cup (women) and ½ –1 cup (men) (Not allowed for the first three weeks of phase two)	• Beans: kidney, lima, navy, pinto, red, black • Black-eyed peas • Green peas • Butter beans • Chickpeas (garbanzo beans) • Green beans • Lentils • Yams • Sweet potatoes
Cereals (Not allowed for the first three weeks of phase two; cereals must be combined with unsweetened almond milk or unsweetened nonfat coconut milk)	• Old fashioned oatmeal or steel-cut oatmeal (1 serving for women; 1–2 servings for men) • Quaker Oats High-Fiber Instant Oatmeal (plain or cinnamon), 1 packet • Quaker Oat Bran Cereal
Low-Glycemic Fruits ½ cup (Fruit only allowed in the morning)	• Blackberries • Blueberries • Raspberries • ½ grapefruit • Granny Smith apple • Kiwi • Strawberries

Vegetables Serving = at least ½ cup or more (women) and 1 cup or more (men). If desired, you may add Butter Buds, Molly McButter, Smart Balance Butter Burst spray, or spices to your vegetables	• Asparagus • Bell peppers • Broccoli • Brussels sprouts • Butternut squash • Cabbage or sauerkraut • Carrots (limit to ½ cup and eat raw) • Cauliflower • Celery • Collard greens • Cucumbers • Eggplant • Lettuce • Okra • Onions • Spinach • Squash • String beans • Taro • Tomato • Turnips • Watercress • Zucchini

Lean proteins (limit to every three to four days—at each meal and snack)	
Dairy It is best to avoid dairy, but if you must have it, choose nonfat cottage cheese or cream cheese or certain Greek yogurts.	• Cottage cheese, nonfat plain: ½ cup • Cream cheese, fat-free (Philadelphia): 4 tablespoons • Low-fat Greek yogurt, plain or vanilla (must be without fruit, fruit syrup, or honey)
Eggs	• Eggs (pastured or organic preferred): two to three large eggs or one egg yolk with three egg whites

Meats	
Meats Serving = 2 to 6 ounces for women and 3 to 8 ounces for men, depending on lean body mass and activity level (do not deep-fry meats)	• Beef, extra lean (preferably organic or free-range; remove all visible fats): limit total red meat consumption to less than 18 ounces a week • Buffalo, bison, elk, caribou, venison, goat, ostrich • Chicken and turkey (remove skins) • Turkey bacon • Turkey sausage • Fish (cod, flounder, haddock, herring, halibut, mahi-mahi, sea bass, tilapia, perch, snapper, tongol tuna, orange roughy, salmon, trout, sardines, mackerel): choose wild rather than farm raised • Pork* (lean ham, lean pork chops, pork tenderloin, Canadian bacon): limit pork to one to two servings per week • Shellfish* (shrimp, crab, lobster, scallops, oysters, mussels)

* If eating pork or shellfish bothers you for religious reasons, I recommend that you avoid it. However, there is no scientific research to prove that these foods are harmful if you eat moderate amounts of organic, free-range selections that are cooked well.

Healthy fats and oils (two servings per day: one serving for breakfast, 1 serving for lunch, and ⅓ serving with each snack, but none for dinner or evening snack)	
Fats (May use a small amount of Pam spray)	• Almond butter: 2 tablespoons • Almonds: about 18 almonds (1 ounce) • Organic peanut butter: 2 tablespoons • Peanuts: 1 ounce • Pecans: 1 ounce • Cashews: 1 ounce • Avocado, fresh: ½ cup, pureed • Guacamole: ⅓ cup • Hummus: 8 tablespoons or ½ cup • Smart Balance Butter Burst Spray: 5 sprays • Organic extra-virgin olive oil: 1 tablespoon • Cold-pressed peanut oil: 1 tablespoon • High-oleic sunflower oil: 1 tablespoon • Cold-pressed sesame oil: 1 tablespoon • Cold-pressed avocado oil: 1 tablespoon • High-oleic safflower oil: 1 tablespoon • Pumpkin seeds: 2 tablespoons or 1 ounce • Sunflower seeds: 2 tablespoons or 1 ounce • Flaxseeds: 3 tablespoons or 1 ounce
Salad Dressings Serving = 10 sprays Use only spritzers with 1 calorie per spray; limit to 10 sprays	• Balsamic vinaigrette (Wishbone Salad Spritzers Balsamic Breeze) • Ken's Steakhouse Salad Spritzers
PGX fiber	I recommend two to four PGX fiber capsules with 8 to 16 ounces of water before each meal

It is my mission to help you maintain your weight and enjoy a healthier lifestyle and method of eating. Now and forevermore, you will weigh yourself as soon as you get out of bed and empty your bladder. Weigh without clothes. It is very important for you to take your scales with you when you travel.

Any weight gain greater than 2 pounds over your final phase two weight is significant. If this happens, you need to repeat an hCG cycle (phase one) as outlined in chapter 7.

The next lifestyle change involves the incredible benefits of healthy snacking. Once you've moved on to the anti-inflammatory diet, healthy snacking will be an important component of your life. Turn to chapter 9 to learn how the right snacks will help prevent hunger and help you burn more belly fat.

Chapter 9

TREATS
AND CHEATS

THOUGH MANY YEARS have passed, I still remember those carefree days of my youth, sitting around a campfire that lit up the pitch-black sky for miles. On these monthly outings with our Scout troop, everyone loved huddling around the fire and staring at its glow while we talked and enjoyed its warmth against the cool night air. Its glow had an unspoken command: if we wanted to continue enjoying the heat, someone had to stoke the fire during the night. I can remember often waking up, shivering, and walking over to the fire to put more wood on it. Every Boy Scout understood that the more wood you put on the fire, the hotter and longer it burned. If we did this throughout the night, we could wake up warm.

Snacks help fuel your body in a similar way. By consuming "mini-meals" in between your three main meals, you stoke your body's metabolic fires, which enable you to burn more calories throughout the day. If it were just a matter of keeping your dietary fires burning, however, many people would not have weight issues. The problem starts with cravings.

WAGING WAR WITH A SNACK

If you are like many people, at some point during the day you probably experience an overwhelming desire for a particular food—usually something you know you should avoid. On the days when you do not feel like fighting the battle, the craving quickly goes from a thought to a single bite to an all-out binge session. If you're like most people struggling with their weight, afterward you feel guilty, ashamed, and maybe even hopeless over the thought that you are locked into a grueling, never-ending struggle with your appetite.

Sound familiar? I encounter this with patients every day. They may be eating three healthy meals a day, getting regular activity, practicing portion control, and avoiding sodas and sweets. Yet without fail, in the midafternoon or post-dinner hours, it is as if someone flips an appetite switch and all they can think about is food—typically the wrong kind.

The truth is that no matter how many carrots or celery sticks you eat, your cravings are not likely to vanish. But before you put down this book and think that there's no point in fighting, understand this: even though you may not be able to eliminate cravings, you can eventually overcome them. The key is controlling them. And one of the most important and effective ways is by snacking.

Snacking Right

Many people do not understand that a good snack can turn off your appetite and can stop the triggers from setting it off in the first place. And though it seems counterintuitive to some, snacking can help you burn more calories in the process. Researchers have determined that snacking on the right amount of healthy foods, in addition to eating three meals a day, boosts the metabolic rate more than if you only eat three meals each day.[1] Snacking stimulates the body to burn more energy. Eating either a meal or a snack every three to four hours will keep hunger in check as well as boost the metabolic rate.

By now I hope you have caught my emphasis on *quantity* and *quality* when it comes to food, including snacks. It does you no good to eat healthy snacks if you consume too many or too much. According to a survey conducted by the Calorie Control Council, one-third of all adults put "snacking too much" as a main reason their weight-loss efforts had failed.[2] I have had to correct many patients who used the power of snacking as an excuse to essentially add a fourth or fifth meal to their daily intake. Even when they chose healthy foods as snacks, they wound up eating massive portions—and the wrong mixture. This obviously defeats the purpose of a weight-loss plan. Avoiding mountain-sized snacks should be a no-brainer.

Likewise, just because you happen to throw the right amount of something on the fire to prevent it from going out does not mean the fire will necessarily burn longer. You have to throw the right kind of fuel on the fire—or the right kind of snack. Twinkies, Krispy Kreme doughnuts, kettle corn popcorn, and high-sugar granola bars don't count. Each of these is similar to putting hay on a fire; it burns up quickly. Eating the wrong kinds of snacks will usually cause you to crave more high-sugar, processed snacks. In other words, when you habitually down a whole pack of Oreo cookies for a "snack," you fill yourself with the wrong fuel and make it likely you will crave that many again. This is why overweight and obese people can often eat their favorite foods and yet never feel satisfied.

HEALTHY SNACKS

So what makes for a healthy snack to ward off these cravings? The word *diet* conjures up images of things like carrots, celery sticks, and broccoli. Although these are healthy foods, they will definitely not satisfy your appetite or hunger. Trying to restrict yourself to this kind of regimen means you may eventually binge on sugary foods and carbohydrates. The best type of snack food is a mini-meal consisting of healthy protein; a high-fiber, low-glycemic carbohydrate or starch; and some good fat. When mixed together, this food fuel or fuel mixture is digested slowly, causing glucose to trickle into your bloodstream, which controls your hunger for hours.

Five Snack Duds

1. Cookies (even if they're fat free, watch out for those calories and sugar)

2. Granola bars (some pass the test, but most are loaded with sugar)

3. Chips and nachos (fat, fat, fat . . . the bad kind too)

4. Cakes and pastries (tons of calories, lots of sugar and fat, and zero nutrition)

5. Crackers (although few are OK, many are loaded with butter or oil)

Portion control is a key to wise snacking. Select half a serving of either a low-glycemic starch or one serving size of fruit. Then add 1 to 2 ounces of a protein and a third of a serving size of fat. Typically this mini-meal should amount to just 100 to 150 calories for women and 150 to 250 calories for men. Here are a few examples of well-rounded snacks.

Morning or afternoon snack

- A piece of fruit (fruit can be eaten whole or blended into kefir); 6 ounces of coconut, low-fat plain kefir, or yogurt; 5 to 10 nuts; and 1 scoop of vanilla or chocolate protein powder

- 2 tablespoons of guacamole with raw carrots or celery and 1 to 2 ounces of turkey, chicken, or roast beef (meat optional)

- 2 tablespoons of hummus with raw carrots or celery (4 inches in diameter) and 1 to 2 ounces of sliced chicken or turkey (meat optional)

- 1 to 2 wedges of Laughing Cow Light cheese and 1 to 2 ounces (for men), 1 ounce for women of smoked salmon or tongol tuna (meat optional)

- Half a cup of nonfat cottage cheese, a piece of low-glycemic fruit, and 5 to 10 nuts

- A small salad with a 1 to 2 ounces of sliced turkey and 2 tablespoons of avocado; use a salad spritzer (meat optional)

- A bowl of broth-based vegetable or bean soup with 1 to 2 ounces of boiled chicken

- Carrots or celery, 1 teaspoon almond butter or peanut butter, and ¼ cup of nonfat cottage cheese

- A protein smoothie made from protein powder (1–2 scoops) mixed with 8 ounces of low-fat coconut milk, almond milk, or low-fat plain or coconut kefir (option: dilute the coconut milk, almond milk, or kefir by reducing it to 4 ounces and combining with 4 ounces of filtered water or spring water)

Bar None

Countless dieters go wrong by assuming a snack bar is healthy just because the words *healthy*, *protein*, or *low-carb* appear on the wrapper. In fact, finding a tasty, healthy, balanced snack bar is a challenge. Most are either loaded with sugars and carbohydrates or with fats—and should be classified as cookies. Others are loaded with low-quality proteins but have no healthy ratio of complex carbohydrates, good fats, and fiber. In addition, many use soy for protein, which is not the best for weight loss. Very few have adequate fiber; most leave you craving more. So you end up eating two, three, or the whole box to satisfy your craving.

Unfortunately, no perfect snack bar exists. The four I recommend, only on occasion but not every day, are the Jay Robb JayBar, any FitSmart bar, and the Nutiva Hemp Chocolate Bar. The best snack option is still a mini-meal using real food rather than a man-made substitute. However, keep a healthy snack bar in your purse or briefcase for emergencies. Most of these snack bars can be found in health food stores instead of supermarkets. Avoid snack bars sold in most supermarkets—they are high in sugar and refined carbs. Remember, as with every meal, a good fuel ratio for a snack bar is 40 percent low-glycemic carbs, 30 percent healthy fats, and 30 percent quality proteins, along with 3 to 5 grams of fiber per bar.

Be sure to take two or three PGX fiber capsules with a 16-ounce glass of water with your snack. And remember you can add as many non-starchy vegetables as you want. To top it off, I recommend a cup of green or black tea, using natural stevia as a sweetener.

Evening snacks

- Protein drink
- Lettuce wraps
- Salad with lean meat
- Vegetable soup with lean meat

A HEALTHY SNACK STASH

Make sure you have cleaned out all the junk food, chips, crackers, candies, cookies, ice cream, sodas, and high-sugar beverages from your refrigerator, freezer, pantry, and cabinets. The second part of that equation is keeping these places stocked with healthy snacks, including plenty of low-glycemic fruits, seeds, nuts, hummus, low-fat cheese, avocados, baby carrots, celery, and the like. Get a large bowl and fill it with fruits, especially high-fiber fruits such as Granny Smith apples, kiwi, grapefruit, and all types of berries. Keep different deli meats, such as nitrite-free free-range turkey, chicken, lean roast beef, lean ham, and organic nitrite-free beef jerky, in the refrigerator. I also recommend always having a supply of low-fat coconut and almond milk; nonfat, low-fat, or part-skim cheese, such as Laughing Cow Light cheese; nonfat cottage cheese or nonfat cream cheese; nonfat or low-fat plain or vanilla Greek yogurt; and kefir and coconut kefir. All of these are simple items that you can take on the go.

Good Fruits

A Brazilian study found that women who ate three small apples or pears a day lost more weight on a low-calorie diet than those who didn't add fruit to their diet. Because of the high fiber in these fruits, those fruit-eating females also ate fewer calories.[3]

In addition, buy different nut butters, including almond butter, cashew butter, and natural peanut butter. Have a supply of hummus, avocado, guacamole, seeds and nuts, tomatoes, and cucumbers readily available so you can mix these with different salads and salad spritzers. (Most salads now come in ready-to-serve bags.) For those who often face time restrictions, you can also have a stash of healthy snack bars mentioned earlier in this chapter. Keep green, black, or white tea; stevia; and a supply of lemons and limes around as well.

Along with making sure you stock your home with these easy snack items, be prepared at work and other places. I tell my female patients to always carry a healthy snack in their purses, such as a Hemp Chocolate Bar, a small bag of nuts, a Granny Smith apple, baby carrots in a resealable plastic bag, and PGX fiber capsules. Keep items that are not perishable in your desk drawer at work. Always be prepared by having plenty of healthy snacks at home, in the office, and on the road. Don't forget: it is important to get snacks that you truly enjoy. Otherwise you won't bother.

CONTROLLING SEVERE CARB
AND SUGAR CRAVINGS

I have already discussed how our digestive system uses up sugary foods and processed carbohydrates within a couple of hours. This rapid digestion causes appetite triggers to repeatedly fire, raising your blood sugar and insulin levels and ultimately causing you to store fat and gain weight. Even obese people have a natural sense for this process; they know firsthand how quickly a sugar high fades away, only to be met by another irresistible craving for more.

Yet what do you do if your cravings for these high-sugar, starchy items are natural? What happens when the different snacks I listed above do not turn off your tremendous cravings for these foods? This is usually the case for those who have low serotonin levels in the brain. Serotonin is an important neurotransmitter that calms us down, helps us control our appetites, and gives us an overall feeling of well-being. Having a low serotonin level causes us to crave sugary foods, chocolates, carbohydrates, and starches.

For many individuals this is a serious matter, not just an occasional hankering for a chocolate bar. These people typically have been under long-term chronic stress and have probably had high cortisol levels for years. They may be chronic low-carb dieters, or they battle insomnia, depression, or PMS. Some may also be compulsive eaters and bingers. They typically think about food all the time and are emotional eaters who use food as comfort whenever they feel lonely, bored, sad, anxious, or angry. Women are more prone to fall in this category than men because the female brain produces 50 percent less serotonin than the male brain.[4] This is also why women often go through "carbohydrate withdrawals" more often. A duo of scientists researched this physiological need for serotonin in some people and identified the problem. Judy Wurtman, PhD, and her husband, Dr. Richard Wurtman—both neuroscientists at the Massachusetts Institute of Technology—discovered that, among other things, there were carbohydrate snacks that could boost serotonin levels in the brain.[5] These could ultimately decrease cravings and help control the appetite. I recommend 5-hydroxytryptophan (5-HTP) for sugar- and starch-craving patients if they have some of the symptoms of low serotonin levels mentioned above. I usually recommend 50 milligrams of 5-HTP one to three times a day or at bedtime. If you are on an antidepressant medicine, consult your doctor before taking 5-HTP. (See Appendix B.)

SEROTONIN-BOOSTING SNACKS

Once you find the snack that works best for you, I recommend that you put the snack in a resealable plastic bag. Then carry the bag in your car, purse, or briefcase. By eating this snack at the specified times, you will control your appetite and boost your metabolic rate. I also recommend consuming 16 ounces of water and two to three PGX fiber capsules before eating a snack. Whether you deal with low serotonin levels or not, snacks are a powerful thing for any successful weight-loss program. They help control the appetite, which is one of the strongest forces that can come against your efforts to lose pounds and keep them off. In cases of low brain serotonin levels, this force can seem overwhelming. Let me assure you, it is not. With simple preparation you will soon learn it can be easily managed—even to the point of becoming routine.

Chapter 10

EATING OUT AND
GROCERY SHOPPING

T HE NATIONAL RESTAURANT Association estimates Americans spend 49 percent of their food
budget at restaurants. It's no wonder that for 2011
the association forecast the industry would reach a
record $604 billion in sales and achieve positive growth
after a three-year-long downturn.[1] Clearly, eating out is
a way of life for millions of American families. Snap-
shots of families enjoying home-cooked meals over the
dinner table in the 1950s and 1960s have faded into
history. Today's meals occur at places like Burger King,
Subway, or McDonald's. The ones taken at home are
most likely of everyone gathered around a take-out box.

With America's fast-paced lifestyle, many parents feel
they do not have time to prepare family meals, leading
to an unhealthy reliance on fast-food restaurants. Meanwhile singles or couples without children at home have
discovered that eating out regularly is easier and may be
more economical. Still, there are ways to avoid settling
into a convenience-food rut. All of us will eat out from
time to time—it is part of modern life. However, if you
hope to control your weight, there are basic principles

you must understand when deciding what dishes to order at restaurants and which foods to cook at home. The key, in both cases, is knowing how to make wise, healthy choices.

THE TWIN CULPRITS

There are two main reasons why eating out sabotages weight-loss efforts. The first is simple: most restaurants serve unhealthy foods. Restaurant owners know that flavor sells. To get repeat customers and generate word-of-mouth, they accentuate flavor through unhealthy cooking. It's the principle of supply-and-demand: the public demands tasty, high-calorie, high-fat meals—and that's what they get. To add insult to injury, these meals are usually loaded with sugars, salt, and high-glycemic carbohydrates. And they are low in fiber, fruits, vegetables, and nutritional value. Individuals who consistently eat at such restaurants struggle to shed any weight.

Don't buy the hype, either. Reacting to health advocates and headlines about obesity problems, in the summer of 2011 the restaurant association announced its "Kids LiveWell" initiative. Introduced at nineteen chains, among its criteria is offering a children's meal of 600 calories or less and other items with limited calories, fat, sugars, and sodium, and a serving of fruit, vegetables, or other sensible options.[2] While it is admirable that some restaurants are responding to the obesity crisis, don't think that means you can eat anything on their menus.

In addition, recognize that you can count calories all day long at other meals, but if you continue to dine out regularly without learning healthy habits, your weight-loss efforts *will* fail. It will be like training to compete in the Olympics but showing up for the trials without a clue of how to run a specific event. Unless you come prepared each time you set foot in a restaurant, you will repeatedly blow your chances.

The second reason eating out can sabotage weight loss is huge portion sizes. Simply put, high-calorie foods plus out-of-control portion sizes equal weight gain and obesity—the equation our culture generally follows.

You can be different by learning to dine out but not succumb to the feasts that tempt you. This starts with understanding portion sizes. Since most servings are large enough to satisfy two people, my wife and I share entrées while ordering a side salad and extra vegetables. The majority of restaurants are willing to bring our food on separate plates. If you and your partner cannot agree on an entrée, order separately and ask your server to put half the portion in a to-go box before bringing the food to the table.

WALKING THROUGH A RESTAURANT MEAL

Many weight-loss patients ask for advice on ordering the right dishes. When I ask about what they usually eat, I often discover they are making wise choices. Most understand they need to apply the principles I mentioned previously—dividing their plate as they do at home and being mindful of eating a proper mix of foods.

However, what I also learn is they either forget about smaller portions or overlook all the extras they consume. For the sake of simplicity, let's walk through a typical dinner so you get an idea of how to apply wise principles to restaurant meals.

The first question every server asks is, "What would you like to drink?" Don't automatically reply Pepsi or Coke. You can save hundreds of calories by avoiding sugar-laden sodas or sweet tea, which are liquid candy. Alcohol is another questionable choice. When consumed before or early in your meal, it rapidly enters your bloodstream and can affect judgment and food selections. You are more likely to overeat or be lax about eating unhealthy foods.

This is not to say you can never enjoy a glass of regular (not dessert) wine. Just make sure you drink it with your entrée and limit yourself to one glass. If you are a tea drinker, order unsweetened tea with a wedge of lemon or lime. Sparkling water or bottled water is another excellent choice. Take two to four PGX fiber capsules with 16 ounces of unsweetened tea or water.

After you order a drink, it's best to refuse the bread all together. Your first temptation is usually bread and butter. Who among us hasn't tried to alleviate hunger pangs by going through three small loaves of bread spread with butter or dipped in olive oil before the salad even hits the table? Also, if you want an appetizer, choose one with vegetables and meats such as a shrimp cocktail. Avoid any that are deep-fried, high in starch and fats (i.e., quesadillas or corn bread), or bread based. Again, it's best to avoid most appetizers.

Remember to order your salad with the dressing on the side and with no croutons, cheese, or fattening side items. It's best to bring your own salad dressing spritzer.

Add a bowl of broth-based vegetable or bean soup to fill yourself up before the entrée.

The entrée is your most important dietary decision. Meat, fish, or poultry should be baked, broiled, grilled, or stir-fried in a minimum amount of oil. Avoid anything deep-fried or pan-fried. Always ask if your meat selection will be fried; if so, ask if it can be cooked another way. If the menu does not list a meat serving's ounces, ask your server. If more than 4 ounces (for women) or 6 ounces (for men), ask the server to put at least half in a to-go box. Naturally you should avoid or significantly limit sauces, cheeses, or gravies. If you must have them, ask that the chef put them in a small side dish. Also request that vegetables be steamed (unless you prefer them raw) *without* any butter or oils.

There is usually an ample supply of starches—which is why most eating establishments' calorie counts are sky-high. Keep in mind the low-glycemic rule, and don't ruin a balanced meal by indulging in butters or fatty oils. If you're a potato fan, remember that baked potatoes are high glycemic. Instead choose a sweet potato if possible—and keep it to the size of a tennis ball. When facing limited options, take two or three PGX fiber capsules or drink a glass of water mixed with fiber to lower the starch's glycemic value.

The final (and greatest) temptation is dessert. Be prepared; servers aren't doing their job unless they try to entice you with a tray crammed with mouth-watering treats. The more desserts they sell, the higher the tab and the larger the tip. How to avoid this? Before the meal ends, ask the server to not bring out the dessert tray. If you don't, you will be confronted with a sales presentation trying to persuade you that the double-fudge chocolate sundae with whipped cream *just can't be* that bad.

If you still choose a dessert, avoid downing the dish solo. Share it, and only take a few bites. Savor those bites. After all, your taste buds aren't asking for a mound of dessert—they just want some flavor.

Careful Planning

One of the easiest ways to avoid disaster is preparation, which helps avoid unhealthy foods and overeating. The first rule of thumb: never go out to eat when you feel ravenous. I guarantee that you will eat too much of the wrong foods. Before leaving home, eat a large Granny Smith apple or a healthy snack, such as a Nutiva Hemp Bar. This will pre-fill your stomach and help prevent overeating.

In addition, plan what and where you will eat *before* leaving. When people don't know where they're going and arrive at whatever restaurant they stumble across, they usually have no idea what they will order. If you hope to lose weight, these are bad moves. I suggest patients also plan an early dinner, usually between five and six o'clock. By doing this, they will usually not have to wait for a table (helping to avoid a grumbling stomach) and will finish early enough to burn off some calories before going to bed.

If you know you will spend time with friends or family at a restaurant, plan on practicing mindful eating. Share an entrée with your spouse. Slow down while eating, and chew every bite thoroughly, putting your fork down between bites. All these "little" things go a long way in controlling hunger and weight. Not only will your brain get the message sooner that you are satisfied, but also you will be able to relax and enjoy conversation with loved ones.

Choices of Restaurants

We all have our favorite types of restaurants. Unfortunately most of us developed those preferences long before we considered healthy eating. For some that is not a problem, since their favorite serves healthy dishes. For others, it may present a challenge. Regardless of preference, it is important to know how to make healthy menu selections. Here's how.

Fast-food restaurants

I link the rise of obesity in our nation with the emergence of fast-food restaurants. Their most popular choices are high in fats, salts, high-glycemic carbohydrates, and calories, and the sodas are loaded with sugar. Not only do fast-food restaurants' "supersized" portions trigger weight gain, their processed ingredients ensure that people get caught in a cycle of junk-food cravings. Have you ever wondered why most fast-food restaurants have rock-hard plastic seats? The seats, colors, lighting, air, and other factors are designed to get you to eat in a hurry, leave, and make room for other customers. Then, when you're hungry again in a few hours, they hope you will return.

In the event you can't avoid them, try the following at

a typical hamburger-oriented chain: Instead of ordering a double cheeseburger (around 500 calories), large french fries (500 calories), and a large soda (about 300 calories), try a grilled chicken sandwich or a small hamburger. Throw away the top and bottom bun, and squeeze your burger between two napkins to remove excess grease. Cut the hamburger in half and then place both halves of the meat between two lettuce leafs. Instead of mayonnaise and ketchup, choose mustard, tomato, onions, and pickle. Now you have a much healthier burger without excessive, high-glycemic carbohydrates.

You can also order a small salad and ask for fat-free dressing (or use just a small portion of a regular packet). For a drink, order unsweetened iced tea or a bottle of water. Instead of french fries, order a baked potato when available, using only one pat of butter or 2 teaspoons of sour cream.

If you eat at a sub shop, imitate Jared Fogle, the Subway guy who lost more than 240 pounds by making the right choices. Choose turkey, lean roast beef, and chicken instead of bologna, pastrami, salami, corned beef, or other fatty selections. Choose a 6-inch sub on the smaller bottom of the bun and not the top portion. Use plenty of vegetables, and top with vinegar; avoid or go easy on the oil. It's best to further cut calories by ordering it in a lettuce or pita wrap.

At fast-food chicken restaurants, instead of fried, choose rotisserie or baked chicken. Peel off the skin and pat the chicken dry with a napkin. Drain the liquid from the coleslaw, and do not eat the biscuit or potatoes.

If you're craving pizza, go easy; it is one of the worst

weight-loss saboteurs. Before diving into a slice, eat a large salad. Then have only one slice of pizza, sticking to thin or flatbread crust. Choose chunky tomatoes and other veggies as toppings. Avoid pepperoni and other highly processed meat toppings, and ask for half the cheese (the same way many ask for double cheese). Finally, use a napkin to remove excess oils from the cheese.

Buffet-style restaurants

If you hope to lose weight, it is wise to avoid buffet-style restaurants. Most are loaded with fried foods, unhealthy starches, and an assortment of fattening desserts. They offer too much food and too few wise choices, with the exception of some salads and vegetables.

There are a few alternatives for the all-you-can-eat variety, such as a healthier Sunday buffet at a sit-down restaurant. Many offer beautiful salads, fruits, vegetables, smoked salmon, lean meats, fish, and grilled or baked chicken. Just watch out for high-calorie foods, including desserts. Still, they typically have enough healthy options. Start with a large salad (but go easy on the dressing or use a spritzer) and fruit, followed by an entrée with plenty of vegetables. If you get a dessert, limit yourself to a couple bites.

Steak houses

These are common choices for special occasions. The portion sizes are so large (including football-sized baked potatoes) that two people can share one entrée. Remember to avoid indulging in the bread beforehand,

and choose a lean, petite fillet, grilled or baked chicken, grilled fish, or shellfish. Choose steamed vegetables and a large salad (again, with dressing on the side or in a spritzer). While a shrimp cocktail on occasion is fine, beware of béarnaise sauce, hollandaise sauce, gravies, creamed vegetables, cheese sauce, and au gratin dishes. All are loaded with fat.

Italian restaurants

Even at my favorite restaurants I have to watch out for eating too much pasta and indulging in high-fat, creamy sauces. I advise starting with a soup—minestrone, pasta fagioli, or broth-based tomato—and a large salad. Limit bread and olive oil, which has 120 calories per tablespoon. Good entrée options include grilled chicken, fish, shellfish, veal, and steak. Avoid fried or Parmesan dishes, such as chicken or veal Parmesan. Ask for your vegetables to be steamed, and avoid the pasta or have it cooked al dente. Don't overdo it on the pasta; the amount should be about the size of a tennis ball. Avoid fat-filled creamy sauces, cheese, and pesto sauce.

Mexican restaurants

Mexican food is usually loaded with fat and starches, starting with the tortilla chips. Since these deep-fried treats are full of calories, ask your server to remove them from the table. Instead, tortilla soup without the chips and black bean soup are good appetizers. In addition, be wary of entrées smothered in melted cheese, which automatically increases the fat count.

Despite these hazards I enjoy Mexican food, usually

choosing fajitas with chicken. You can also get beef or shrimp, and the meat is usually stir-fried or grilled, meaning it is healthier. Add such ingredients as salsa, onions, lettuce, beans, and guacamole. Beware of over-eating cheese and sour cream—avoid them if possible, since restaurants rarely serve nonfat varieties.

As for beans, choose red or black but not refried, since they are high in fat. Avoid the rice. If a salad is available, enjoy a large one before your entrée. Avoid the tortilla, and make your fajita with lettuce wraps.

Chinese, Thai, or Vietnamese restaurants

These are usually good choices, provided your meat or seafood is baked, steamed, poached, or stir-fried. Steaming is usually the healthiest method. Some Chinese restaurants stir-fry their meat in excessive oil, using as much as a half a cup. Instead of fried rice or fried noodles, choose brown rice. Remember that eating white rice is like eating sugar. Sometimes restaurants will allow you to substitute a serving of rice with vegetables. If not possible, take two or three fiber capsules, and don't eat more than a tennis-ball-sized serving of rice. Avoid sweet and sour, batter-fried, or twice-cooked food (which is high in fat and calories) and oily sauces (i.e., duck). For an appetizer you can choose wonton or egg drop soup instead of deep-fried egg rolls.

The downside to many Chinese restaurants is that many use monosodium glutamate (MSG) to enhance the flavors of main dishes. I recommend finding one that doesn't use MSG or is willing to not use it on your dishes. MSG has numerous potential reactions. The most common is stimulating your appetite, causing you to become hungry again in a couple hours. More importantly, MSG can lead to severe headaches, heart palpitations, and shortness of breath. (For more information on MSG, refer to my book *The Seven Pillars of Health*.)

Japanese restaurants

Japanese food is usually low in fat and features many vegetables. Unfortunately it is also high in sodium, primarily because of abundant use of soy sauce. An easy solution to this is to add only a small amount of additional soy sauce (if any) to your food. Sushi is fine; some restaurants prepare it with brown rice. Steamed vegetables, vegetable soups, and salads with dressing on the side are also good choices. Seafood, chicken, and beef can be cooked teriyaki style. Fish can be steamed or poached. Be cautious with eating too much rice, and avoid fried foods.

Indian restaurants

Many Indian foods contain large portions of ghee (clarified butter) or oil, so it's best to find a restaurant willing to limit the amount they use on your dish. Tandoori-cooked (roasted) or grilled fish, chicken, beef, and shrimp are good choices. Avoid deep-fried foods and sauces, such as marsala sauce and curry sauce, which are high in fat. If you must have them, get them in a small side dish. Also, it's best to avoid the breads—a major element of Indian food. If you have any, however, choose bread that is baked *nan* instead of the fried *chapatis* bread.

French restaurants

Although French cooking is usually high in fat, most French restaurants serve smaller portions than standard restaurants. In recent years a new type of French cooking, called nouvelle cuisine, has emerged that is generally lower in fat. Whichever style you choose, select meats or fish that are grilled, steamed, or broiled. Avoid foods baked in cheese or creamy sauces, or have the sauces served in side dishes and eat sparingly. Most French restaurants serve an abundance of vegetables and fruit; make them the majority of your meal. Because these restaurants are renowned for their pastries and desserts, it's best to avoid them or to be mindful if you sample a dessert. Savor a few bites and share the remainder.

Family-style restaurants

Foods at these restaurants are typically high in fats; the main courses are often fried. The vegetables are usually loaded with gravy, butter, or oil. Good choices include baked or grilled chicken, turkey, or beef with steamed vegetables. Vegetable soup and a salad (dressing on the side) also make good choices. Avoid the large dinner rolls and butter and fried side dishes. Choose beans, such as lima, pinto, or string beans. If you must have gravy, get it on the side and eat it sparingly. Though raised on Southern cooking, I have learned I can enjoy the foods without all the gravies and fried options.

GROCERY SHOPPING TIPS

Now that you have learned more about making wise restaurant choices, you need information about healthy shopping. Many of my patients start eating programs on the wrong foot. They sabotage early weight-loss efforts by stocking their refrigerators, freezers, and pantries with junky, processed, sugary, and fatty foods.

As with restaurants, shopping in grocery stores takes advance planning to avoid common marketing traps. Like restaurants, supermarkets are carefully designed to entice you to buy certain foods—and lots. The cardinal rule is simple: *eat before you shop.* If you arrive hungry, you will be too likely to grab too many comfort foods.

It is no coincidence that when you walk into a grocery store you get hit by the aroma of freshly baked pastries, pies, and cookies. If the slightest bit hungry, your resolve will quickly dissolve. It isn't just you, either. Every decision at the grocery store affects everyone in your family. You can shape your children's future simply by what you stock at home.

Every trip should start at home by making a list of only the items you need. This makes you less prone to impulse purchases. Try to list exact brands and amounts; if confronted with a sale price for a high-calorie, high-fat alternative, you will be more likely to stand your ground.

PERIMETER SHOPPING

Let's start our trip by looking at what's on the perimeter. The healthiest food choices are usually located on the outer aisles. This is where you want to start filling your cart with smart buys.

Fruits and vegetables

As I explained earlier, half of your plate at lunch and dinner should consist of vegetables. You will want to spend an adequate amount of time in this section to choose a variety of vegetables and low-glycemic fruits. Unfortunately most people always buy the same fruits and vegetables and rarely try anything different. If trying to lose weight, you will likely be eating more vegetables than in the past, so I challenge you to try new things. In the process you may discover a favorite new vegetable or fruit.

My wife, Mary, purchases prepackaged organic vegetables and salads, which can cut preparation time in half. Besides eating them raw, Mary and I often steam, stir-fry, or grill our vegetables. To enhance their flavor, we add spices, seasonings, or such condiments as Molly McButter or Butter Buds. Both of these alternatives are fat and cholesterol free and low in calories (5 calories a teaspoon).

As you're shopping, choose a variety of colors of fruits and vegetables. Each color offers unique, protective phytonutrients and antioxidants. Phytonutrients play a significant role in preventing various cancers and heart disease. Because there are literally thousands—all have tremendous health benefits—I urge people to try to eat all the colors of the rainbow each day.

Remember farmers' markets too. These are seeing a resurgence, thanks to younger people wanting fresh, organic, and locally grown produce. In the United States most food you find on a grocery store shelf has traveled an average of more than fifteen hundred miles from the farm that produced it.[3] Farmers' markets offer an alternative to long-distance shipping and are located nationwide. Often they offer a wider variety of produce.

Another great source is community-supported agriculture (CSA). This allows you to buy organic produce directly from local farmers. CSAs create a sense of community by connecting farmers and consumers, in addition to establishing a mutually supportive relationship and an economically stable farming operation. You can find more information at www.nal.usda.gov/afsic/pubs/csa/csa.shtml.

Meats and fish

Still on the perimeter, meats are usually found at the back. Always choose lean cuts; I advise free-range, range-fed, organic, or drug- and hormone-free meat and poultry. Most cattle are grain fed, which means fattier meat. Ask the butcher to trim off all visible fat. You can also purchase lean roast beef at the deli.

Since most luncheon meats are fatty, high in sodium, and contain nitrites and nitrates, which form cancer-causing nitrosamines, look for low-sodium, low-fat, and nitrite- and nitrate-free luncheon meats. Chicken and turkey are good choices that you can purchase as luncheon meats or entire portions free of nitrites and nitrates. Chicken strips make good fajitas and are good in a stir-fry dish.

Wild salmon, sardines, grouper, and tilapia make

great seafood choices. Choose wild fish instead of farm-raised fish, since the latter typically have higher levels of chemicals, including PCBs and heavy metals. Although tuna has moderate amounts of mercury, small tuna or tongol tuna is generally low in mercury and available in many health food stores. You may eat shellfish (shrimp, crab, lobsters, and oysters) occasionally, but make sure it is cooked well.

You can also eat lean pork (ham, pork chops, roast, or tenderloin) occasionally. However, make sure the butcher trims off visible fat. Avoid sausage because of its high fat content. While bacon is high in saturated fat, certain nitrite-free turkey bacon is acceptable (and delicious). You may also choose Cornish hens, veal, lamb, duck, bison, or elk—all typically low in fat.

Dairy

With the exception of those allergic to dairy or who are lactose intolerant, most people enjoy dairy. However, not all dairy is healthy. If available, always opt for organic. If too expensive, you can choose regular fat-free or low-fat items. I recommend organic low-fat or fat-free plain kefir or yogurt, as well as small amounts of low-fat or fat-free milk and cheese. But do not eat dairy daily, but instead rotate eating small amounts every three to four days. Other wise choices include fat-free cottage cheese, ricotta cheese, part-skim milk cheese, and Laughing Cow Light. Choose organic butter over regular, but use it sparingly; it is still high in fat.

Also, if you experience nasal congestion from eating dairy foods, eliminate all cheese. If that doesn't help, try low-fat or nonfat goat milk products instead. Use caution and moderation with dairy, and do not get in the habit of eating it every day.

You're Getting Colder

Next comes the frozen foods section. If fresh vegetables are unavailable, choose frozen. Since they are frozen at their ideal ripeness, these chilled veggies may contain more nutrients and antioxidants than fresh—especially those transported across the country, a process that can cause them to lose nutrients.

Frozen dinners

The average American cooks and eats a frozen meal about six times a month; as a nation we spend almost $6 billion per year on frozen meals.[4] For these and other reasons, frozen dinners take up more shelf space than any other type of frozen food. I prefer my patients eating fresh food instead of frozen dinners. The key is finding tasty selections that satisfy but are still healthy and do not sabotage weight loss.

One of the most important factors in finding a good product is learning how to read the nutrition label. Many light frozen dinners contain less than 300 calories, 8 grams of fat or less, and are not filling for most people (especially men). Yet dinners that are more filling are often overflowing with fat, sodium, and starch. This is just another reason to avoid most frozen dinners.

Criteria for choosing a healthy frozen dinner

- Men can consume up to 550 calories, while women should aim for 250 to 400. (Most men can choose two low-calorie items if they are each 275 calories or less.)

- Choose meals with less than 15 grams of fat and less than 7.5 grams of saturated fats. Make sure that they contain no trans, hydrogenated, or partially hydrogenated fats.

- Choose meals with 600 milligrams or less of sodium.

- Look for at least 3 grams of fiber; 5 to 10 is preferred. You may supplement this with fiber capsules or fiber powder to reach 10 grams.

- It should have preferably 40 grams of carbohydrates or less, and it's always best to avoid wheat, cornstarch, and white rice.

- It should contain at least 15 grams of protein.

- It should contain less than 15 grams of total sugars, including corn syrup and malt dextrin.

I know these guidelines can seem overwhelming, but it is important to make healthy choices by reading nutrition facts on the label. Many people choose low-calorie frozen dinners that meet various criteria but do not satisfy their hunger. That is why it is good to augment frozen dinners with a large salad and some steamed vegetables or a bowl of broth-based vegetable or bean soup.

Some of my favorites are certified organic dinners from Helen's Kitchen. Other good choices include Healthy Choice, Kashi, South Beach Living, Lean Cuisine, or Smart Ones. Below is a sampling:

Healthy Choice

- Traditional Turkey Breast With Gravy and Dressing—300 calories, 550 mg sodium, 4 g fat, 42 g carbs, 21 g protein, 6 g fiber

- Sesame Chicken—230 calories, 600 mg sodium, 6 g fat, 35 g carbs, 12 g protein, 3 g fiber

- Rosemary Chicken With Sweet Potatoes—180 calories, 500 mg sodium, 2.5 g fat, 26 g carbs, 12 g protein, 5 g fiber

- Roasted Chicken Verde—230 calories, 500 mg sodium, 3.5 g fat, 35 g carbs, 14 g protein, 3 g fiber

- Honey Balsamic Chicken—220 calories, 540 mg sodium, 3.5 g fat, 34 g carbs, 12 g protein, 5 g fiber

- Portabello Parmesan Risotto—220 calories, 590 mg sodium, 4 g fat, 35 g carbs, 9 g protein, 4 g fiber

Kashi

- Chicken Pasta Pomodoro—280 calories, 470 mg sodium, 6 g fat, 38 g carbs, 19 g protein, 6 g fiber

Lean Cuisine

- Chicken Florentine Lasagna—290 calories, 650 mg sodium, 6 g fat, 37 g carbs, 21 g protein, 3 g fiber

Smart Ones (Weight Watchers)

- Picante Chicken and Pasta—260 calories, 480 mg sodium, 4 g fat, 32 g carbs, 23 g protein, 4 g fiber

Most frozen dinners—even some listed above—do not contain the perfect fuel mixture for weight loss since they are usually higher in carbohydrates and sugar content and low in protein. Therefore don't eat them for every meal or even once a day. Limit them to one or two times per week—or less.

Caution: Entering the Inner Aisles

You need to exercise caution when entering the inner aisles of grocery stores. Many products are enticing and attractively packaged yet loaded with sugars, fats, and calories. Here you will find processed foods, junk foods, and countless tempting high-calorie synthetic foods.

Cereals

Choose steel-cut oatmeal in place of processed oatmeal. Add some cinnamon and berries, cook them in the oatmeal, and sweeten with stevia. I have found that by eliminating most grains, especially wheat and corn, most patients will start losing belly fat. Eating oatmeal two to four days is acceptable.

Pastas and rice

Avoid pasta and rice for the most part to lose belly fat, but eventually small amounts of brown or wild rice or al dente brown rice pasta are allowable.

Breads

It is best to avoid bread to lose belly fat, but millet bread may be rarely eaten once every three to four days. It tastes better if toasted. Eventually, when most belly fat is gone, you may choose to eat Ezekiel bread or other sprouted breads in moderation.

Oils

My favorite oil is extra-virgin olive oil and other monounsaturated fats including avocados, almonds, cashews, hazelnuts, pecans, macadamia nuts, peanuts, sunflower seeds, pumpkin seeds, and nut butters. Also, chia seeds, flaxseeds, and flaxseed oil are other favorites since they contain anti-inflammatory omega-3 fats. So are wild salmon, sardines, and anchovies. If you choose others, make sure they are cold-expeller pressed vegetable or nut oils such as extra-virgin olive oil and high-oleic safflower and sunflower oil. However, even healthy oils are still loaded with calories—approximately 120 calories per tablespoon. Go easy on the oil.

You now have completed most of your grocery shopping and should have avoided purchasing many foods that sabotage weight-loss efforts. Your pantry and refrigerator will now contain the foods that will satisfy your appetite and enable you to lose weight.

Chapter 11

SUPPLEMENTS THAT SUPPORT WEIGHT LOSS AND BURN BELLY FAT

EVER WATCH *The Red Green Show?* The offbeat series features Steve Smith as Red Green, who interacts with his hapless nephew, Harold, and a cast of wacky characters at Possum Lodge. Even though they stopped filming new episodes in 2006, reruns still air on Canadian television, the Comedy Network, and various Public Broadcasting System channels. Red is always looking for shortcuts to car repairs, home improvements, or unusual inventions, usually winding up with fractured, rib-tickling results. His solution to every problem: duct tape. He calls it the handyman's secret weapon.

Too many people are equally naive when it comes to fixing their weight problems. Instead of duct tape, they think either a certain diet pill will do the trick or that downing the latest health drink a few times a day will suddenly make the pounds disappear. Many people are looking in vain for a magic pill that will enable them to eat anything they want, never exercise, and still lose weight. To quote an old cliché, "It ain't gonna happen."

Sure, things like amphetamines may appear to do the trick for a while. They suppress appetite and accelerate metabolism, allowing you to temporarily lose weight. However, the adverse reactions can be extreme: insomnia, nervousness, palpitations, headaches, arrhythmias, angina, heart attack, stroke, hypertension, hostility, aggressive behavior, and addiction, to name a few. Amphetamines may also worsen depression and anxiety. When you stop taking them, the reactions can be as severe as those I just listed. One common withdrawal response among users: regaining the weight they lost—and more.

SEARCHING FOR THE MAGIC BULLET

For years doctors, researchers, pharmaceutical companies, and nutritional companies have hunted for "The Pill to End All Diets." In the early 1990s researchers believed they had found it through combining two appetite suppressants—phentermine and fenfluramine. Known as fen-phen, this combo effectively suppressed appetite and became a hit. Individuals lost weight and kept it off as long as they continued on the medication. Studies revealed stunning results: on average, most users lost almost 16 percent of their body weight in just eight months. As an example, that correlates to a 200-pound person losing an impressive 32 pounds.

Willing to Pay

Sales of weight-loss drugs in the United States have surpassed the $1 billion mark, crossing that threshold in the fall of 2010.[1]

As you would expect, these results stimulated the formation of weight-loss clinics across America, where doctors prescribed this miracle pill combo. Yet after only a few years of use, a small percentage of users died of an extremely rare disease called primary pulmonary hypertension (PPH). This affected several patients out of one hundred thousand; about half of them eventually required a heart-lung transplant to survive. To their credit, drug companies immediately pulled the two fenfluramine drugs, Pondimin and its derivative, Redux, off the market. However, authorities found phentermine to be relatively safe.

A few years later supplement companies once again believed they had found the magic pill, combining the herb ephedra with caffeine. This also proved to be a powerful formula for turning down the appetite and burning fat. Again, over the years both the effectiveness and the safety of ephedra were called into question. Ephedra has been linked to severe side effects, including arrhythmias, heart attack, stroke, hypertension, psychosis, seizure, and even death. To show what a major concern this is, consider a single statistic from the National Institutes of Health: products containing ephedra comprise less than 1 percent of all dietary supplement sales. Yet those products are responsible for an incredible 64 percent of adverse reactions from dietary supplements.[2]

Due to safety concerns, in 2004 the Food and Drug Administration (FDA) banned ephedra products in the United States. Although a federal court later upheld the ban, companies wiggle around it by selling extracts that contain little or no ephedrine. And some related herbs, such as bitter orange (citrus aurantium) and country mallow, remain on the market. Like ephedra, bitter orange supplements have been linked to stroke, cardiac arrest, angina, heart attack, ventricular arrhythmias, and death. These products are potentially lethal. I do not recommend them unless taken under the direction and close monitoring of a knowledgeable physician.

Among other herbs of concern is aristolochia, which is found in some Chinese herbal weight-loss supplements and may not even be listed as an ingredient. Aristolochia is a known kidney toxin and carcinogen in humans. There are also products containing usnea (usnic acid), a lichen for weight loss that can cause severe liver toxicity. In addition, some Brazilian diet pills have been found to be contaminated with amphetamines and other prescription drugs.[3]

Alli and Hydroxycut Side Effects

Alli, one of the most common over-the-counter diet pills, may cause bowel changes in its users. These changes, which result from undigested fat going through the digestive system, may include gas with an oily discharge, loose stools or diarrhea, more frequent and urgent bowel movements, and hard-to-control bowel movements.

Hydroxycut products were recalled in May 2009 after reports of deadly liver failure and disease in individuals who took the products to lose weight. According to the *World Journal of Gastroenterology*, an ingredient in Hydroxycut from a fruit called *Garcinia cambogia* caused the liver disease and failure.[4]

Meant to Supplement, Not Replace

I hope by now you understand that for every supposed magic weight-loss pill, potential dangerous side effects loom close by. Unfortunately these often remain undiscovered until thousands—if not millions—of hopeful dieters have taken them. A few users have died. Let me remind you, the foundation for weight loss is simple: a healthy dietary plan and regular physical activity. The primary reason people are overweight or obese is too much calorie intake and too little physical activity. Period.

A weight-loss supplement is a nutritional product or herb intended to assist your healthy eating and activity plan with the ultimate goal of losing weight. A supplement comes alongside; it does not replace. Do not be deceived by crafty marketing that promises otherwise. Weight-loss and dietary supplements are not subject to the same standards as prescription drugs or medications sold over the counter. They can be marketed with only limited proof of safety or effectiveness.

However, there are a number of safe and fairly effective dietary supplements that look promising for weight loss. Each supplement has its own unique mechanism of action for weight loss, with some having more than one. I have categorized these beneficial and proven supplements into the following categories:

- Thermogenic agents (fat-burning agents)
- Appetite suppressants
- Supplements to increase satiety

- Supplements to improve insulin sensitivity
- Supplements to increase energy production

There are many causes of obesity; however, aging is one of the most common. This is because of a decrease in energy expenditure associated with aging. According to scientists, this may cause the body to store 120 to 190 excess calories daily. This may mean an extra 13 to 20 pounds of extra body fat a year.[5] Since there are many causes of obesity, I recommend adding a few safe nutritional supplements that work through different mechanisms, such as thermogenic agents, natural appetite suppressants that increase satiety, supplements that increase insulin sensitivity, and energy products. In treating hypertension, heart disease, diabetes, and other diseases, doctors add different medications with different mechanisms of action because when they are combined, their action is synergetic and more powerful. We now have safe, natural supplements that work by different mechanisms in helping individuals lose weight. Combining these will usually increase their effectiveness.

Green Is Good

A study found that after three months of taking green tea extract, overall body weight declined 4.6 percent while waist circumference decreased by nearly 4.5 percent.[6]

THERMOGENIC (FAT-BURNING) AGENTS

The term *thermogenic* describes the body's natural means of raising its temperature to burn off more calories. More specifically, thermogenesis is the process of triggering the body to burn white body fat, which is the kind of fat we often accumulate as we age—the kind we typically see in overweight or obese people. Thermogenic agents, then, are fat burners that help to increase the rate of white body fat breakdown. Fortunately most unsafe thermogenic agents have been pulled off the market.

Green tea

Green tea and green tea extract are my favorite weight-loss supplements. Green tea has been used for thousands of years in Asia as both a tea and an herbal medicine. It has two key ingredients: a catechin called epigallocatechin gallate (EGCG) and caffeine. Both lead to the release of more epinephrine, which then increases the metabolic rate. Ultimately green tea promotes fat oxidation, which is fat burning. It also increases the rate at which you burn calories over a twenty-four-hour period.

An effective daily dose of EGCG is 90 milligrams or more, which can be consumed by drinking three or four cups of green tea a day. Do not add sugar, honey, or artificial sweeteners to it, though you may use the natural sweetener stevia.

Italian researchers created a green tea phytosome by combining green tea polyphenols with phospholipids, which caused a significant increase in the absorption of the polyphenols, including EGCG. A clinical trial involved one hundred significantly overweight subjects. Half the group received the green tea phytosome in a dose of two 150-milligram tablets daily. Both groups were placed on a reduced-calorie diet (1,850 calories a day for men and 1,350 calories a day for women). However, after forty-five days the control group lost an average of 4 pounds and the green tea phytosome group lost an average of 13 pounds, about triple the control group. After ninety days the control group lost an average of 9.9 pounds; the green tea group lost 30.1 pounds. The green tea phytosome group saw a 10 percent decrease of waist circumference, but the control group only realized a 5 percent reduction.[7] In addition to drinking green tea, I recommend 100 milligrams of green tea supplement three times a day. (See Appendix B.)

Green coffee bean extract

A placebo-controlled study reported in January 2012 that green coffee bean extract produced weight loss in 100 percent of overweight participants. For twenty-two weeks participants were given 350 milligrams of green coffee bean extract twice a day. They did not change their diets, averaging 2,400 calories per day, but they did burn 400 calories a day through exercise. The results included:

- Average weight loss of 17.6 pounds, with some subjects losing 22.7 pounds

- Average body fat decrease of 4.4 percent with some subjects decreasing by as much as 6.4 percent

- Average BMI decrease of 2.92 points

- A majority of participants (85.7 percent) were able to maintain the weight loss after completing the study

- No side effects[8]

So how does it work? The key phytonutrient in green coffee bean extract is chlorogenic acid, which has the ability to decrease the uptake of glucose, fats, and carbohydrates from the intestines and thus decrease the absorption of calories. It also has positive effects on how your body processes glucose and fats, and it helps to lower blood sugar and insulin levels.

Drinking coffee doesn't give you the same effects, and it can also cause sleeping problems for some. But because of roasting, most of the chlorogenic acid in coffee is destroyed. (Light roasted coffee has more chlorogenic acid than dark roasted coffee, but the amount is still too low.)

By comparison, the extract is much better. Green coffee bean extract should contain 45 percent or more of chlorogenic acid. In addition, green coffee bean extract only contains about 23 milligrams of caffeine per serving vs. a cup of coffee with over 100 milligrams of caffeine. That's why in addition to—or in place of—drinking coffee, I recommend taking 400 milligrams of green coffee bean extract thirty minutes before each meal. (See Appendix B.)

Meratrim

Meratrim is a blend of two plant extracts that has been shown in two independent placebo-controlled studies to significantly reduce body weight, BMI, and waist measurement within eight weeks when used with a diet and exercise plan. The studies show that 400 milligrams of Meratrim twice a day, thirty minutes before breakfast and thirty minutes before dinner, achieved these results by interfering with the accumulation of fat while simultaneously increasing fat burning.[9] (See Appendix B.)

THYROID SUPPORT

All obese patients should be screened for hypothyroidism, including the blood tests TSH, Free T3, Free T4, and thyroid peroxidase antibodies to rule out Hashimoto's thyroiditis, the most common cause of low thyroid. If a patient has low body temperature (less than 98 degrees), they most likely have a sluggish metabolism and may have sluggish thyroid function.

It's especially important to optimize the Free T3 blood level to improve the metabolic rate. The normal range of T3, according to the lab I use, is 2.1 to 4.4. I try to optimize the T3 level to a range of 3.0 to 4.2 by using both Levothyroxine (T4) and Liothyronine (T3). I can sometimes optimize the T3 levels with natural supplements including Metabolic Advantage or iodine supplements. (See Appendix B.)

I also commonly perform a lab test to see if a patient is low in iodine before starting iodine supplements. According to the American Thyroid Association, 40 percent of the world's population is at risk for iodine deficiency.[10]

APPETITE SUPPRESSANTS

These supplements generally act on the central nervous system to decrease appetite or create a sensation of fullness. Although some medications in this category include risk-prone phenylpropanolamine (found in such products as Dexatrim), I have found a few safe, natural supplements that are extremely effective appetite suppressants.

L-tryptophan and 5-HTP

L-tryptophan and 5-hydroxytryptophan (commonly known as 5-HTP) are amino acids that help the body to manufacture serotonin. Serotonin assists in controlling carbohydrate and sugar cravings. L-tryptophan and 5-HTP also function like natural antidepressants. If you are taking migraine medications called triptans or SSRI (selective serotonin reuptake inhibitors) antidepressants, you should talk with your physician before taking either supplement. The typical dose of L-tryptophan is 500 to 2,000 milligrams at bedtime. For 5-HTP it is typically 50 to 100 milligrams one to three times a day or 100 to 300 milligrams at bedtime. Serotonin Max is an excellent supplement that helps boost serotonin levels naturally. (See Appendix B.)

What's the Point if a Pill Can Do It?

Marketing researchers have found that the more proven a drug is to be effective at shedding pounds, the more lax the efforts of the user at continuing to eat well and exercise. Those who take prescription or over-the-counter diet pills are more likely to engage in eating junk food and living a sedentary lifestyle.[11]

L-tyrosine, N-acetyl L-tyrosine, and L-phenylalanine

L-tyrosine, N-acetyl L-tyrosine, and L-phenylalanine are naturally occurring amino acids found in numerous protein foods, including cottage cheese, turkey, and chicken. They help to raise norepinephrine and dopamine levels in the brain, which then helps decrease appetite and cravings and improves your mood. (SAM-e is another amino acid that helps raise norepinephrine and dopamine levels.) Doses of L-tyrosine, N-acetyl L-tyrosine, and L-phenylalanine may range from 500 to 2,000 milligrams a day (sometimes higher), but they should be taken on an empty stomach. I prefer N-acetyl L-tyrosine for most of my patients since the body absorbs it better than L-tyrosine or L-phenylalanine. I typically start patients on 500 to 1,000 milligrams of N-acetyl L-tyrosine, taken thirty minutes before breakfast and thirty minutes before lunch. I do not recommend taking any of these supplements in late afternoon because they may interfere with sleep.

Fiber Away!

In addition to PGX, another great fiber for weight loss is glucomannan, made from the Asian root konjac. Glucomannan is five times more effective in lowering cholesterol when compared to other fibers such as psyllium, oat fiber, or guar gum. Because it expands to ten times its original size when placed in water, it is a great supplement to take before a meal to reduce your appetite as it expands in your stomach, but you should take it with 16 ounces of water or unsweetened black or green tea.

SUPPLEMENTS TO INCREASE SATIETY

Fiber supplements and foods high in fiber increase feelings of fullness by using several different mechanisms. Fiber slows the passage of food through the digestive tract, decreases the absorption of sugars and starches into the stomach, and expands and fills up the stomach—turning down the appetite. Although the American Heart Association and the National Cancer Institute recommend 30 grams or more of fiber each day, the average American only consumes between 12 and 17 grams.[12]

When it comes to losing weight and managing blood sugar levels, a little fiber goes a long way. One study found that consuming an extra 14 grams of soluble fiber each day for only two days was associated with a 10 percent decrease in caloric intake.[13] Soluble fiber supplements significantly increase post-meal satisfaction and should be taken before each meal to assist in weight loss. Soluble fiber lowers the blood sugar, slowing down digestion and the absorption of sugars and carbohydrates. This allows for a more gradual rise in blood sugar, which lowers the glycemic index of the foods you eat. This helps to improve the blood sugar levels.

PGX Fiber

PGX, short for PolyGlycoPlex, is a unique blend of highly viscous fibers that act synergistically to create a much higher level of viscosity than the individual fibers alone. The viscosity is the gelling property. PGX absorbs hundreds of times its weight in water over one to two hours and expands in the digestive tract, creating a thick gelatinous material. It creates a feeling of fullness, stabilizes the blood sugar and insulin levels, and stabilizes appetite hormones.

PGX lowers blood sugar after eating by about 20 percent and lowers insulin secretion by about 40 percent. Researchers have found that higher doses of PGX can decrease appetite significantly. PGX works similar to gastric banding and has fewer gastrointestinal side effects than other viscous dietary fibers. However, start slowly or you may develop gas.

Taking soluble fiber before meals helps you feel satisfied sooner and usually decreases the amount of calories you consume. One study showed that 7 grams of the supplement psyllium before a meal decreased hunger and food intake while stabilizing blood sugar and insulin levels. In fact, special fiber blends, such as glucomannan, xanthan, and alginate (PGX), appear to be more effective than taking a single type of soluble fiber. In another study, participants took six PGX capsules before every meal. By the end of the three-week study, those taking the PGX had decreased their body fat by 2.8 percent.[14]

The fiber that I prefer for weight-loss patients is PGX. I start with one capsule, taken with 8 to 16 ounces of water before each meal and snack, and then gradually increase the dose to two to four capsules until patients can control their appetite. Always take PGX with evening meals and snacks. (See Appendix B.)

SUPPLEMENT TO INCREASE
ENERGY PRODUCTION

L-carnitine is an amino acid that functions as a transporter of energy by shuttling fatty acids into the mitochondria, which act as our cells' energy factories by burning fatty acids for energy. In essence, L-carnitine helps our bodies turn food into energy. Humans synthesize very little carnitine, so we may need to supplement from outside sources. This applies especially to obese and older individuals, who typically have lower levels of carnitine than the average-weight segment of the population. As you might expect, individuals with insufficient carnitine have a greater difficulty burning fat for energy.

Milk, meat, fish, and cheese are good sources of L-carnitine, while mutton and lamb are also rich in this amino acid. In supplement form, I recommend combining L-carnitine with lipoic acid, PQQ (pyrroloquinoline quinone), and a glutathione-boosting supplement to increase energy production. A glutathione-boosting supplement will help quench free radicals in the mitochondria, including hydroxyl and hydrogen peroxide, which in turn helps to increase ATP production and one's energy. PQQ is a powerful antioxidant that protects the mitochondria from oxidative damage and actually stimulates the growth of new mitochondria. The mitochondria are, figuratively speaking, the energy factories in our cells that produce ATP, which is our energy currency. Some cells such as the myocardial cells (heart muscle cells) have thousands of mitochondria, and other cells such as fat cells have very few mito-chondria. L-carnitine, acetyl-L-carnitine, lipoic acid, PQQ, as well as glutathione-boosting supplements are all important to protect the mitochondria, grow new mitochondria, quench oxidative damage to the mito-chondria, and increase energy production. One form of carnitine, acetyl-L-carnitine, is also able to cross the blood brain barrier and increase the energy of brain cells. This has numerous neuroprotective benefits and helps to increase neurotransmitters in the brain. It also protects brain cells from the effects of stress.

Overall I recommend taking a combination of L-carnitine and acetyl-L-carnitine, lipoic acid, PQQ, and a glutathione-boosting supplement. By increasing your energy, you will be more likely to exercise regu-larly and burn more fat. The best time to take these sup-plements is in the morning and early afternoon (before 3:00 p.m.) on an empty stomach. If you take them any later, these supplements can impair your sleep. (See Appendix B.)

Also, green tea supplements and N-acetyl L-tyrosine help to increase your energy.

OTHER COMMON SUPPLEMENTS TO ASSIST WITH WEIGHT LOSS

Irvingia

Irvingia is a fruit-bearing plant grown in the jungles of Cameroon in Africa. Irvingia gabonensis helps to resensitize your cells to insulin. It appears to be able to reverse leptin resistance by lowering levels of C-reactive protein (CRP), an inflammatory mediator. In a double-blind study, 102 overweight participants received 150 milligrams of Irvingia or a placebo twice a day for ten weeks. At the end of the period the Irvingia group lost an average of 28 pounds and the placebo group just 1 pound. The Irvingia group also lost an average 6.7 inches from their waistline and decreased total body fat by 18.4 percent. They also had a 26 percent reduction of total cholesterol, a 27 percent decrease in LDL (bad cholesterol), a 32 percent decrease in fasting blood sugar, and a 52 percent decrease in CRP.[15]

It is believed that Irvingia has the ability to enable one to lose weight by simply lowering CRP levels, which in turn lowers leptin resistance. Leptin is a hormone that tells your brain you've eaten enough and that it is time to stop. It also enhances your body's ability to use fat as an energy source. One also needs zinc, 12 to 15 milligrams a day, which is present in most comprehensive multivitamins, in order for leptin to function optimally.

Unfortunately, because of Americans' sedentary lifestyles and highly processed, high-glycemic food choices, many overweight and obese patients have acquired resistance to leptin. As a result, this hormone no longer works properly in their bodies. Similar to insulin resistance, leptin resistance is a chronic inflammatory condition that contributes to weight gain and belly fat. It is critically important to follow the dietary program that I have outlined in this book, which is also an anti-inflammatory diet. Simply decreasing inflammatory foods enables most to start losing belly fat and also allows leptin to function optimally.

I have been using Irvingia with patients since 2008 and have seen remarkable improvements. The generally recommended dose is 150 milligrams of standardized Irvingia extract, twice a day, thirty minutes before lunch and dinner.

The hoodia controversy

Hoodia is a South African plant similar to a cactus that may help suppress the appetite. Initially used by tribal leaders to enable them to go on long journeys without getting hungry, various sources cite thousands of years' worth of Bushman history to verify its effectiveness. Although these tribal hunters obviously have not conducted scientific studies to prove hoodia is an effective appetite suppressant, one 2001 clinical study by a company called Phytopharm found individuals who consumed the plant ate 1,000 fewer calories a day than those who didn't take hoodia.[16] One of the company's researchers, Richard Dixey, MD, explained that hoodia contains a molecule that is ten thousand times more active than glucose.[17]

However, there is a catch. When news of this supposed miracle supplement hit the headlines, dozens (if not hundreds) of companies started marketing hoodia—without having any actual hoodia in their products. The result was that more hoodia was "produced" in a single year than in all of African history—highly unlikely, to say the least. Even today it is possible that much of what is sold in the United States either contains ineffective hoodia variations or no hoodia. So be wary of falling for marketing schemes with this substance.

In Summary

While some questionable products are on the market, there are a variety of safe, effective over-the-counter dietary supplements for weight loss. Some people may find that incorporating a combination of these into their eating and activity plan works even better. Others may not need to take any supplements. Most of my overweight and obese patients have found that drinking green tea or taking green tea phytosome, certain amino acids (such as Serotonin Max and N-acetyl L-tyrosine), and PGX fiber supplements before each meal and snack (especially in the evening) helped them shed pounds.

If you continue experiencing problems controlling your appetite or struggle with food cravings, decreased energy, or insulin resistance, you will likely require one or more of the supplements I just reviewed. The same goes if you do not feel full or satisfied after a meal or if you have low hormone levels. However, I remind you what I said earlier: supplements are just supplements, not magic pills. Excess weight was years in the making, so it won't suddenly vanish. The good news is you no longer have to be duped by wonder-working, flab-busting, "as seen on TV" promises. Armed with the right eating and activity plan, you *can* shed the weight.

Chapter 12

THE IMPORTANCE
OF ACTIVITY

E XERCISE. DOES THAT word fill you with dread and visions of boredom, fatigue, and your tongue hanging out as you gasp for air? If you hate working out, you are not alone. Even big-name celebrities who are known for their ultra-fit bodies and sex appeal disdain it. Singer and actress Janet Jackson says, "I hate working out—and hate is a strong word, but I cannot stand working out."[1] Bruce Willis, known for his tough-guy roles in numerous action-adventure flicks, admits, "I'm lazy, I hate working out, I only do it for films and I think of it as work."[2]

Nor is Willis the only Hollywood star with an aversion to exercise. Actress Katherine Heigl, best known for her Emmy Award–winning performances on *Grey's Anatomy,* says, "If I wasn't in this industry, I wouldn't work out. But I have hips and a butt and everything that goes along with that, including cellulite."[3]

From the world of athletics, listen to tennis star Serena Williams: "I hate working out more than anything, but I have to—when I'm running, I think about how much I want to win. That's the only thing that keeps me going....I guess everyone has to find that one thing that encourages them and just think about it the entire time you're working out. But I have to be honest, I hate going to the gym. I don't like running. I hate doing anything that has to do with working out."[4]

The one person you might have expected to champion exercise was fitness buff Jack LaLanne, who died in January of 2011 at age ninety-six. Even the legendary workout master once said, "I hate exercise, but I love the results."[5] Such quips illustrate our love-hate relationship with exercise. In particular we dread taking the time out of our already cramped schedules for it. What other explanation is there for all the late-night TV infomercials about time-saving exercise gadgets promising pounds will "instantly" fall off if we use their product? We always want the quick solution.

As a result, two-thirds of all Americans are not physically active on a regular basis. Less than half get less than the recommended amount of exercise. Sadly a full 25 percent—a quarter of the population!—get absolutely no exercise.[6] The leading reason, according to almost every survey conducted, places time at the top of its list of excuses.[7] People rationalize they are just too busy to exercise. According to the CDC, the average adult, age eighteen to sixty-four, needs 150 minutes (2.5 hours) a week of moderate aerobic activity and two or more days a week of muscle-strengthening activity.[8] A recent study found that women over forty-five years of age need 60 minutes of moderate exercise a day to prevent weight gain as they aged, even with consuming a normal diet.[9]

WHAT'S IN A WORD?

While you may not think you have the time, exercise is essential for good health. That applies to every human being—especially anyone hoping to shed weight. You can restrict your diet and eat less than your daily requirement. Yet without burning off calories through physical activity, you have only completed half the weight-loss equation. After working with thousands of overweight and obese individuals, I have discovered that almost without exception, they struggle with a perception of exercise. And, it all comes down to that single word: *exercise.*

Marathon Burn

To burn off the 1,510 calories in a Quiznos large Chicken Carbonara, you'd have to expend the same calories it takes to bike across the state of Delaware (thirty miles).[10]

For many, *exercise* conjures up the same negative feelings as *diet.* Those who are overweight or obese think of exercise in terms of pain, sweating, humiliation, embarrassment, and anxiety. They may visualize themselves in a health club surrounded by people with perfect bodies, a physical education instructor testing their lack of physical capabilities, or an overbearing coach from their youth. Because this word often stimulates dread, I use a different one: *activity.* To some, this seems a bit silly. It's just a word, after all—what difference could substituting one word make? Isn't it still referring to the same thing?

I cannot explain why this works, but it does. *Activity* seems less intrusive; it doesn't trigger emotional symptoms or anxiety. For most overweight or obese individuals, it is safe and nonthreatening. It does not overwhelm them with thoughts of time commitments, discipline, or early-morning alarm clocks.

It is up to you whether you adapt a change of vocabulary. However, the bigger issue you cannot overlook is that both a change of diet and regular activity are crucial for weight loss. Plain and simple, the reason why people successfully lose weight and keep it off is because they are physically active.

THE PERKS OF REGULAR ACTIVITY

In case you needed a reminder, here are some of the many benefits that come with regular activity:

- It decreases the risk of heart disease, stroke, and the development of hypertension.

- It helps prevent type 2 diabetes.

- It helps protect you from developing certain types of cancer.

- It helps prevent osteoporosis and aids in maintaining healthy bones.

- It helps prevent arthritis and aids in maintaining healthy joints.

- It slows down the overall aging process.

- It improves your mood and reduces the symptoms of anxiety and depression.

- It increases energy and mental alertness.

- It improves digestion.

- It gives you more restful sleep.

- It helps prevent colds and flu.

- It alleviates pain.

- And the favorite reason among overweight and obese people...it promotes weight loss and decreases appetite.

Don't use Hollywood stars or fitness gurus as an excuse to justify a lack of activity. When push comes to shove, you must do your part and get moving regularly. This takes courage. If it didn't, everyone would do it. You must take the offensive to battle, remembering that obesity is a scourge that can weaken and damage other organs in your body.

The Natural Weight-Loss Supplement

There is no better way to complement a weight-loss dietary and supplement program than physical activity. How does it help? The ways are as plentiful as the many benefits I just listed. First, it helps raise the metabolic rate during and after the activity. It enables you to develop more muscle, which raises the metabolic rate all day—even while you sleep. It decreases body fat and improves your ability to cope with stress by lowering the stress hormone cortisol.

Such activity also raises serotonin levels, which helps reduce cravings for sweets and carbohydrates. It assists in burning off dangerous belly fat and improves your body's ability to handle sugar. Finally, regular physical activity can even help control your appetite by boosting serotonin levels, lowering cortisol, and decreasing insulin levels (which can also decrease your chances for insulin resistance).

Strength in Years

In 2004 Connecticut resident George Brunstad became the oldest man to swim the English Channel when he crossed the twenty-five-mile stretch at age seventy. Though he swam an extra seven miles due to strong currents, Brunstad completed the grueling journey just a minute shy of sixteen hours. Just as admirable was the former pilot's underlying purpose for swimming, which was to let people know about a ministry his church sponsors in Haiti.[11]

There are numerous enjoyable activities to choose from; for example, cycling, swimming, working out on an elliptical machine, dancing, and hiking. Sports such as basketball, volleyball, soccer, football, racquetball, tennis, and squash are all considered aerobic. Pilates, ballroom dancing, washing the car by hand, working in your yard, and mowing the grass qualify too—anything that raises the heart rate enough to burn fat.

A great aerobic activity is brisk walking, although for diabetic patients with foot ulcers or numbness in the feet, walking is not the best activity. In its place they should try cycling, an elliptical machine, or pool activities while inspecting the feet before and after activity. If you can walk, to enter your target heart rate zone, walk briskly enough so that you cannot sing and slowly enough so that you can talk. Following this formula is one reason that I recommend people find an activity partner to talk with them as they walk. (Skeptics might say that misery loves company.)

Here are a few other tips to get you started:

- Choose something that is fun and enjoyable. You will never stick to any activity program if you dread or hate it.

- Wear comfortable, well-fitting shoes and socks.

- If you are a type 1 diabetic, you will need to work with your doctor in order to adjust insulin doses while increasing your activity. Realize that exercising will lower your blood sugar; this can be potentially dangerous in a type 1 diabetic.

MUSCLES, METABOLISM, AND AGING

Everyone wants to look young and fit forever. That's particularly true in the United States, where we plaster buff, sculpted, trimmed, toned, and youthful bodies all over magazine covers, TV ads, and movie screens. Great looks hide the reality that adults typically lose ½ to 1 pound of muscle tissue every year after the age of twenty-five, meaning our bodies naturally progress toward more fat and less muscle. That isn't the greatest news for those overloaded with fat. However, such a realization can be a driving force to shape up. The more muscle mass, generally the higher your metabolic rate and the more calories you will burn at rest. For each pound of muscle mass that you either gain or do not lose, you will burn between 30 and 50 calories a day.

I will never forget the patient I saw years ago during residency. The star running back on a high school football team, he had fractured his left thigh. Part of the reason he played running back was the power in his legs. Not surprisingly, his thighs were extremely muscular. Before, he said, he had been able to leg press more than 1,000 pounds for ten repetitions. Because of his injury, though, this athlete had to wear a full leg cast for approximately two months.

When we removed the cast, we were shocked at how much his left leg had atrophied. Measuring his thighs showed a 32-inch circumference around his mid-right thigh; his left checked in at a mere 24 inches. In only two months inactivity had cost this young man 8 inches of muscle. A similar process occurs with most adults, though not as quickly. Yet if you are inactive, your muscles are slowly melting away. Your metabolic rate is decreasing, and muscle tissue is (typically) being replaced with fat. Many people do not notice because the size of their arm or leg remains the same, when in fact it is simply a case of fat replacing muscle tissue— similar to the marbling of meat.

This is particularly true for women. A woman's metabolism typically begins to decrease at age twenty at a rate of about 5 percent per decade. To understand this, let's use the example of an average fifty-year-old female—I'll call her Sarah. Since her late twenties Sarah's weight has slowly increased from around 120 pounds to her current weight of 150. During those years she gained 30 pounds of fat while losing 15 to 30 pounds of muscle. That may sound like it averages out, except when you consider the corresponding drop in metabolic rate.

At twenty Sarah could eat 2,000 calories a day and maintain her 120-pound frame. At the age of fifty, if she eats 2,000 calories a day, she will most likely gain weight because of this lost muscle tissue. Why? For each pound of muscle tissue lost, your metabolic rate decreases 30 to 50 calories per day. So in addition to losing 15 pounds of muscle, Sarah lost the ability to burn 450 to 750 more calories a day.

Can you see why maintaining or gaining muscle mass is so crucial? Muscle does not just look better than fat; it is essential for maintaining a healthy body. The only way to keep muscle intact is to use it and strengthen it, which means increasing your activity level. When you remain inactive, you put yourself in a body cast—so to speak—as your metabolic rate nosedives and you slowly morph into a fat magnet.

RECOMMENDED AMOUNT OF ACTIVITY

Once I have persuaded patients they need more activity, their next question is: "How much do I need?" Unfortunately no universal number applies. There are numerous factors involved in engaging in activity to lose weight, starting with the heart.

Every activity either requires or can be performed at different levels of intensity. Given that, it makes sense that every person hoping to lose weight has an ideal intensity at which he or she should work out. This is called your target heart rate zone, which generally ranges from 65 to 85 percent of your maximum heart rate.

To calculate the low end of this zone, start by subtracting your age from 220. This is your maximum heart rate. For example, for someone forty years old the formula is:

220 − 40 = 180 beats per minute

Multiply this number by 65 percent to find the low end of the target heart rate zone:

180 x 0.65 = 117 beats per minute

To figure out the high end of the zone, multiply maximum heart rate by 85 percent, or:

180 x 0.85 = 153 beats per minute

So, if you are forty, you should keep your heart rate between 117 and 153 beats per minute when exercising. However, that is quite a wide range, which prompts the next question: Which end of the zone do you aim for to lose weight? Experts have debated this ever since the "target zone" idea came into being many years ago. To find the answer, let's look at the types of activity that push the heart to these two extremes.

BURNING FAT WITH AEROBIC ACTIVITY

The word *aerobic* means "in the presence of air or oxygen." Aerobic activity is simply movement that strengthens the lungs and the heart. It involves steady, continuous movements that work large muscle groups in repetitive motion for at least twenty minutes. The key point for weight loss with aerobic activity is to maintain a moderate pace, which triggers your body to burn fat as its preferred fuel.

One of the most common workout mistakes I see among overweight people is their tendency to jump on a treadmill and run as hard as they can for as long as possible. They intend to burn off more fat by doing this, but in the long run (pardon my pun) they won't. Sprinting, running, or jogging at high intensity for so long you are short of breath actually makes you burn less fat as fuel. For inactive individuals who are just starting to work out, it's also the quickest way to burnout.

Not Just Nervous

Fidgeting or getting up from your seat frequently can cause you to burn an additional 350 calories a day—which amounts to 36 pounds lost in a year![12]

Remember, aerobic means with oxygen; therefore, the activity you choose must be of moderate intensity for your body to use oxygen in order to burn the fat as fuel. When you exercise to the point that you are severely short of breath, you are no longer performing aerobically. Instead you have shifted to an anaerobic activity, which means activity without oxygen. Anaerobic activity burns glycogen—stored sugar—as primary fuel instead of fat. When you run out of glycogen and have not eaten for a while, you may begin breaking down muscle tissue and burning muscle protein as fuel. (Notice that I haven't yet mentioned burning fat.) Many marathoners and triathletes burn a significant amount of muscle as fuel, which is often why they remain so lean.

If you are overweight and aim to burn primarily fat, you need to work out at a moderate intensity of 65 to 85 percent of your maximum heart rate. This is the fat-burning range of your target heart rate zone. As you approach the high end, you near anaerobic activity, which does less good in burning fat. This might be a completely revolutionary idea. If so, it may be a struggle to change. Most people believe that to the hardest worker—meaning the guy who runs the fastest and sweats the most—go the spoils. Not true. If you are overweight or obese, working out at a higher intensity for long stretches may not only sabotage your fat-burning ability, but it may also increase cortisol levels, which can cause more belly fat to accumulate.

When starting any activity program, work out around 65 percent of your maximum heart rate. As you become more aerobically conditioned, gradually increase the intensity to 70 percent of maximum heart rate. After a few more weeks, increase to 75 percent, and so on. You may never be able to work out at 85 percent of maximum rate, especially if you are huffing and puffing. Be sure that as you increase the intensity of your workouts, you remain able to converse with another person. That is a fairly good sign that you are training aerobically and are burning fat. When you are in good aerobic condition, you can start interval training.

Interval Training

High-intensity interval training (HIIT) mixes high-intensity bursts of exercise with moderate-intensity recovery periods, usually for a period of less than twenty minutes. It is used mostly for individuals trying to lose weight.

HOW MUCH?

This brings us back to the original question: how much activity? The Centers for Disease Control and Prevention (CDC) and the National Institutes of Health (NIH) both recommend following the *2008 Physical Activity Guidelines for Americans*, published by the US Department of Health and Human Services. The guidelines recommend that adults need two types of physical activity each week—aerobic and muscle-strengthening. For aerobic activity they recommend two hours and thirty minutes of moderate intensity aerobic activity (brisk walking, water aerobics, riding a bike on level ground, playing doubles tennis, pushing a lawn mower, etc.) every week or one hour and fifteen minutes of vigorous exercise (jogging, swimming laps, riding a bike fast or on hills/inclines, playing singles tennis, playing basketball, etc.) every week. For muscle-strengthening exercise, which I call resistance exercise, they recommend two or more days a week, working all major muscle groups (legs, hips, back, abdomen, chest, shoulders, and arms).[13]

I recommend breaking up the aerobic activity as follows: if you can only do moderate intensity activities, try brisk walking for thirty minutes a day, five days a week. If you can handle more vigorous activity, jog for twenty-five minutes a day, five days a week. Or you can break it down even further: try going for a ten-minute walk, three times a day, five days a week.

A 2004 Duke University study shed some light on this. Over a period of eight months researchers at Duke studied a group of overweight men and women ages forty to sixty-five. Participants were split into four main groups: those who walked twelve miles a week, those who jogged twelve miles a week, those who jogged twenty miles a week, and those who did nothing. None of the groups changed anything about their diets. All exercised at different maximum heart rates. As you might expect, the sedentary group gained weight, added to their waistlines, and upped their body fat percentage. Those who walked twelve miles a week (or thirty minutes a day) did so at 40 to 55 percent of their maximum heart rate. Their results were minimal. The group that jogged this same distance each day kept their heart rates between 65 and 80 percent the maximum rate, meaning they exercised within their target heart rate zone. Though some of their results were similar to the walking group, they did lose more body fat and gained more lean muscle. Finally, those who jogged for twenty miles each week kept within their target heart rate zone and saw by far the best results. On average, the members of this group dropped 3.5 percent of their weight, 3.4 percent of their waist measurement, 4.9 percent of body fat measurements, and added 1.4 percent of lean muscle.[14]

Dog Lovers?

Approximately 60 percent of dog owners do not walk their dogs, simply letting them out in the backyard.[15]

Clearly it pays to be active. The longer you engage in activity at a moderate intensity, the more fat you burn as fuel. I am not suggesting you have to jog twenty miles a week. Still, you can start by choosing enjoyable, fun activities that you and your family can do daily to obtain similar results. Unless you have already been working out, I suggest that you initially set a goal of twenty minutes a day, which may be split into ten minutes, twice a day. (You can do this by simply walking your dog!) Once you have adapted, gradually increase to thirty minutes and eventually forty minutes or more. To minimize soreness, get activity every other day, three days a week, and work up to five or six days a week. And remember, a brisk walk can accomplish almost as much as jogging—provided you maintain 65 to 85 percent of your maximum heart rate.

RESISTANCE EXERCISES

Resistance training usually involves lifting weights to build muscles. These strengthening activities include weight training with free weights or machines, calisthenics, Pilates, resistance band activities, core-specific activities, and balance ball activities. To eliminate the risk of injury, you must maintain good posture and form while performing these exercises. In addition, it is important to learn the correct lifting techniques, the correct range of motion, correct breathing, and the correct speed of the movement in which muscles are being trained.

Thigh Circumference

Thin thighs (less than 24 inches in circumference) are associated with significantly increased risk of death and cardiovascular disease. The risk increases as thigh circumference decreases. This makes it important to maintain a thigh circumference greater than 24 inches.[16]

You should typically perform ten to twelve repetitions per set. When starting resistance training, I recommend only performing one set per activity. This reduces soreness, which is common in beginning any type of strengthening program. As you become better conditioned over time, you can increase to two or three sets per activity for each body part to strengthen and tone muscles. Remember, go slow! Strength training causes microscopic tears in muscle fibers, which eventually causes them to grow stronger and larger. This in turn increases your metabolic rate. Never overdo it and train the same muscles every day; the muscles will not have time to repair and rebuild.

Eventually, after a couple of weeks of strength training, you will be able to increase your workouts to three or four days a week. By following the correct lifting techniques, you will prevent injury, build muscle, and burn fat. I recommend finding a certified personal trainer to teach you this valuable information so you can maximize results. After years of visiting health clubs, I am appalled at the large percentage of people who lift weights incorrectly.

High-Intensity Interval Training

If you've had any success in the past with high-intensity workouts, my guess is that the past few pages of this chapter may have frustrated you. It's hard to convince avid weightlifters and spinning aficionados that moderate-intensity workouts are the best way to burn fat. Most everyone has been trained that the harder you work out and the more you sweat, the more fat you shed. I've already discussed the reasoning for my moderate-intensity preference, but let me explain this a little further before going on.

High-intensity anaerobic workouts obviously have proven value. Not only that, but also studies in recent years have shown that these power cardio routines can be just as effective as longer, moderate-intensity workouts. It's no surprise, then, that the American public, with its usual "faster is better" mind-set, has adopted this as the preferred way to lose fat. However, after helping thousands of overweight and obese individuals to successfully lose weight and keep it off, I believe I have enough credentials to speak on this matter. Let me offer a suggestion for those who have exercised religiously in the past or who become bored quickly with moderate-intensity workouts. Try varying it up once in a while with some high-intensity interval training (HIIT). Notice the word *interval*, however. This is simply alternating between brief, hard bursts of exercise and short stretches of lower-intensity exercise or rest. Various studies in recent years have proven this to be an effective way to improve not only overall cardiovascular health but also your ability to burn fat faster. One study at the University of Guelph in Ontario, Canada, found that following an interval training session with an hour of moderate cycling increased the amount of fat burned by 36 percent.[17] I personally do HIIT three times a week. I warm up on the elliptical machine for five to ten minutes. I then do sixty seconds of high-intensity training with high resistance and as fast as I can. I then decrease the resistance and speed to a lower setting so that I can talk while exercising. I continue this pattern for twenty minutes.

My suggestion is to hold off on HIIT, regardless of your exercise past, until you've consistently done some moderate-intensity activity for several months. I'd rather see you be able to sustain your momentum for the long haul rather than have you burn out, not because of eating the wrong things, but simply because you wanted to sprint to the finish line faster. Be sure to have a physical exam with EKG and or a stress test before starting HIIT.

The Tabata Method

A popular new form of HIIT is Tabata, an exercise regimen created by Izumi Tabata that uses twenty seconds of high-intensity exercise followed by ten seconds of rest, repeated for eight cycles. An alternative routine uses three minutes of warming up, followed by sixty seconds of high-intensity exercise, followed by seventy-five seconds of rest, repeated for eight to twelve cycles.

PUTTING IT ALL TOGETHER

To lose weight, you can literally start your activity program on the right foot. Unless you are physically restricted, walking is the easiest way to stay active. All you need for equipment are some comfortable clothes and a good pair of walking shoes. It's a great way to enjoy the outdoors. Follow my earlier recommendation to find an activity partner, and you can catch up on conversation while he or she holds you accountable with your exercise. Avoid the routine; for variety, go to a park or visit a hiking trail.

Keeping Track

Researchers say that self-monitoring devices, such as a pedometer, heart rate monitor, or even a simple exercise journal can account for a 25 percent increase in successfully controlling your weight.[18]

I believe in monitoring yourself. An excellent way to monitor the steps you walk during the day is by using a pedometer. I urge all my patients to get one and track their step count during the day. Typically a person walks three thousand to five thousand steps a day. To stay fit, set a goal of ten thousand steps, or approximately five miles. To lose weight, aim for between twelve thousand and fifteen thousand steps per day. Other ways to reach this upper target: walking your dog, parking farther out in the parking lot at work or when shopping, and taking the stairs instead of the elevator whenever possible.

Before engaging in any activity, make sure that you have either eaten a meal two or three hours prior or have had a healthy snack about thirty to sixty minutes beforehand. It is never good to work out when hungry; you may end up burning muscle protein as energy—which is very expensive fuel. Remember, losing muscle lowers your metabolic rate.

After you are into the routine of walking approximately thirty minutes, five or six days a week, or you are taking twelve thousand steps a day on your pedometer, you can start resistance training. Before this routine, always do a five-minute warm-up by walking on a treadmill or elliptical machine or riding a stationary bike at low intensity. This increases blood flow to muscles and joints, prepares them for the workout, and significantly reduces the risk of injury.

Once you have warmed up, do a twenty- to thirty-minute workout, using free weights, machines, calisthenics, Pilates, or some other strengthening activity. This burns up much of the glycogen stored in the muscles and liver. Following this, you will be ready for a thirty-minute aerobic workout, such as brisk walking on a treadmill, cycling, or using an elliptical machine or other cardio equipment. This aerobic session allows you to mainly burn fat.

When you are finished with both the strength and aerobic parts of your workout, cool down by doing a low-intensity aerobic activity for another five minutes—just as you warmed up. You may also want to do some stretching after your cooldown.

I recommend a resistance program two to four days a week, working out every other day for twenty to thirty minutes, and an aerobic program five to six days each week for thirty minutes. Always warm up before any activity and cool down at the end. And keep things fun by periodically changing the routine. By varying your activities every month or so, you can shock your muscles into new growth—which means burning more fat. That is a step everyone should want to take.

A Personal Note

FROM
DON COLBERT

G OD DESIRES TO heal you of disease. His Word is full of promises that confirm His love for you and His desire to give you His abundant life. His desire includes more than physical health for you; He wants to make you whole in your mind and spirit as well as through a personal relationship with His Son, Jesus Christ.

If you haven't met my best friend, Jesus, I would like to take this opportunity to introduce Him to you. It is very simple. If you are ready to let Him come into your life and become your best friend, all you need to do is sincerely pray this prayer:

> *Lord Jesus, I want to know You as my Savior and Lord. I believe You are the Son of God and that You died for my sins. I also believe You were raised from the dead and now sit at the right hand of the Father praying for me. I ask You to forgive me for my sins and change my heart so that I can be Your child and live with You eternally. Thank You for Your peace.*

*Help me to walk with You so that I can begin
to know You as my best friend and my Lord.
Amen.*

If you have prayed this prayer, you have just made the most important decision of your life. I rejoice with you in your decision and your new relationship with Jesus. Please contact my publisher at pray4me@ charismamedia.com so that we can send you some materials that will help you become established in your relationship with the Lord. We look forward to hearing from you.

Appendix A

GUIDELINES
AT A GLANCE

EVER ATTEND A social gathering and steadily work your way through the buffet, collecting treats like a vacuum cleaner scoops up dust? You know the drill. It starts with several handfuls of potato, tortilla, or corn chips, stopping to enliven the taste with several spoonfuls of cheese, ranch, or French onion dip. Then it's on to the meat tray for a couple "small" sandwiches of roast beef or turkey, some tomato, a bit of Swiss and perhaps a little Colby, all topped off by a dollop of mayonnaise and a squirt of mustard. Oh, those stuffed mushrooms look good. So do the crab puffs. Those cherry tarts look delicious. And the miniature pecan pies...yummy!

Once you've worked way through the line, chatted with several friends, and rested awhile, it's back for another sampling. Maybe some potato and macaroni salad, another few handfuls of chips, and some other tasty delight you missed the first time. After all, there's so much—you want to try a little bit of everything. All these salt-laden foods call for a thirst quencher too, whether it's a couple 20-ounce soft drinks or a sugary-sweet bottle of Snapple. Before you know it, your belly is protesting about the 2,000 or 3,000 calories worth of food you just crammed into it, even as you're thinking, "Why am I so stuffed? I just had a few snacks."

After reviewing the previous chapters about meal planning and snacks, I hope you have developed a more intentional mind-set toward daily food intake. Fail to take this step, and I guarantee you will fall prey to the office social gathering, family get-together, friend's birthday party, or one of the other calorie-, fat-, and salt-laden temptation-filled occasions that will regularly enter your life. Although I have already covered some of the following, here I want to review some of the recommendations I make to patients who need to lose weight, especially belly fat. I will go into more specifics later on, but to start, here are a dozen basic rules for quick reference. You may want to make a condensed copy of them to post on your desk or carry in your wallet or purse.

- Graze throughout the day (on salads and veggies, not chips and fatty treats).

- As I've said for decades, eat breakfast like a king, lunch like a prince, and dinner like a pauper.

- Eat smaller midmorning and midafternoon snacks, such as protein bars and coconut milk kefir blended with plant, egg white, or whey protein.

- Avoid all simple-sugar foods, i.e., candies, cookies, cakes, pies, and doughnuts.

If you must have sugar, use either stevia, xylitol, Sweet Balance, Just Like Sugar (found in health food stores), or small amounts of coconut sugar or tagatose.

• Drink 2 quarts of filtered or bottled water a day. That includes 16 ounces thirty minutes before each meal, or one to two 8-ounce glasses two and a half hours after each meal. Also, drink 8 to 16 ounces of water upon awakening.

• Avoid alcohol.

• Avoid all fried foods.

• Avoid high-glycemic starches, including wheat and corn products, or at least decrease them dramatically. This includes all breads, crackers, bagels, potatoes, pasta, white rice, and corn. Limit beans, peas, lentils, and sweet potatoes to a half cup, one to two times a day. Avoid bananas and dried fruit.

• Eat fresh, low-glycemic fruits only for breakfast or lunch and occasionally with morning and early afternoon snacks; eat steamed, stir-fried, or raw vegetables, lean meats, salads with colorful vegetables (preferably with a salad spritzer), almonds, and seeds.

- Take fiber supplements, such as two to three capsules of PGX fiber, with 16 ounces of water before each meal and two to three PGX fiber capsules with each snack.

- For snacks, choose bars such as Jay Robb bars and chocolate flaxseed bars. Try to limit these bars to one every day or every other day. These may be purchased at a health food store. (Refer to *Dr. Colbert's "I Can Do This" Diet* for more information.)

- Do not eat later than 7:00 p.m.

General Recommendations

Remember one of the most the important guidelines for weight loss: eat every three to three and a half hours to keep your blood sugar levels stable, and remember to eat healthy, well-balanced snacks. Here are others:

- For meals, choose a lean protein, a low-glycemic carb, and a healthy fat (but make sure you go "carb free" and low fat after 6:00 p.m.).

- For morning snacks, the easiest thing to do is choose a piece of fruit from the Approved Foods chart in chapters 7 and 8. You may also choose from the afternoon snacks listed later in this chapter. As with meals, take two to three PGX

fiber capsules with 16 ounces of water
before or after your snack. It's best to
drink green, white, or regular tea with
your snacks, except for your evening
snack. Remember to drink iced tea or
water since that helps to boost the metabolic rate and will help you lose weight.

• For afternoon snacks, choose any of the
approved snacks from Approved Foods or
a "mini-meal" consisting of a half-serving
of protein, a half-serving of low-glycemic
carbs, and a half-serving of fat. Take one
5-HTP or Serotonin Max if craving sugar
or carbs And remember the PGX fiber
capsules. (See Appendix B.)

• For evening snacks, choose any of the
approved snacks from the Approved
Foods chart or a "mini-meal" (leaving out
the carbs and fats).

• Serving sizes for protein are typically 2 to
4 ounces for women and 3 to 6 ounces for
men.

• Limit red meat intake to a maximum of
18 ounces per week.

• All soups should be low sodium, vegetable
or bean, and broth based, not cream based.

- Use Himalayan or Celtic sea salt instead of regular table salt (in small amounts, less than 1 teaspoon a day).

- It's best to avoid wheat and corn products. I prefer my patients to choose millet bread instead of wheat bread. However, an occasional slice of Ezekiel bread toasted with breakfast or lunch every three to four days is acceptable.

- If desired, you may sweeten foods and beverages with stevia or Just Like Sugar. It is best to avoid artificial sweeteners such as NutraSweet and Splenda.

- You may add a small amount of organic skim milk or low-fat coconut milk to your coffee, if desired.

- If organic foods are too expensive, one option is to at least choose organic for the meat or other protein you consume most often. If you aren't able to buy organic, then choose very lean cuts of meat, peel the skin off poultry, thoroughly wash fruits and vegetables that cannot be peeled, and choose skim milk or 1 percent dairy products and skim milk cheese. (Still, if you can tighten your budget to free up some room for organic or range-fed items, these are the best choices. For meats, Maverick Ranch or Applegate

Farms are good choices. I recommend prepackaged nitrite-free turkey breast, chicken breast, ham, or lean roast beef slices.)

• I recommend that large salads of colorful vegetables, tomatoes, raw carrots, onions, cucumbers, and other vegetables make up the majority of lunches and dinners. Save the salad for your evening meal if you are tired of eating salad at both meals.

• If you choose to make your smoothies with coconut milk, be sure that it only contains 80 calories per cup. (So Delicious is one brand that meets this criteria.) You may have to purchase it from a health food store; however, it is usually available at your local supermarket.

Recommended appliances (all are optional)

To save time on cooking and preparing meals, I recommend:

• George Foreman Next Grilleration Grill
• Vegetable steamer
• Blender
• Toaster
• Convection oven

**Recommended nutritional supplements
(all are optional)**

You can experience weight loss without taking these supplements, but to help you feel full longer, fight cravings, and lose weight faster I recommend the following (more information on these can be found in Appendix B):

- PGX fiber, to help you feel full longer. Begin with one before each meal. Slowly work your way up to two to four capsules until desired feeling of fullness is achieved. It is best taken with 16 ounces of water, except for evening snack. Use only 8 ounces of water with your evening snack since 16 ounces may interfere with sleep.*

- Serotonin Max or 5-HTP to help with food cravings. Take one capsule with your midafternoon snack or with your evening meal or evening snack (if craving sugars or carbs). Or you may take it at bedtime.

- N-acetyl-tyrosine, 500 milligrams, two to three tablets thirty minutes before breakfast and thirty minutes before lunch if hunger and appetite are a problem.

---

* If you can only afford one supplement, PGX fiber is the most important one. The most critical times to take it are before your afternoon snack, evening meal, and evening snack.

- Living Green Tea with EGCG, to help boost metabolism and possibly burn fat faster. Take one capsule three times a day.

- Green coffee bean extract: Take one 400-milligram capsule thirty minutes before each meal.

- Meratrim (Metabolic Lean): Take one capsule twice a day, thirty minutes before breakfast and thirty minutes before dinner.

Recommended protein powders and protein bars (all are optional)

I do not recommend soy-based protein. Instead, try chocolate- or vanilla-flavored whey protein powder, egg white protein powder, or plant protein, which may contain hemp, rice, pea, or plant proteins; this can also be added to oatmeal or cereal. (See Appendix B.)

Dr. Colbert's Healthy Salad Dressing

- ¼ cup organic extra-virgin olive oil

- ¾ cup balsamic vinaigrette (or other vinegar if preferred)

- Juice of ½–1 lemon or lime

- ¼ cup cilantro leaves (optional)

- 1–2 garlic cloves, pressed (or as many as desired for taste)

- Salt and pepper to taste (use Himalayan sea salt)

Mix all ingredients and transfer to a salad spritzer bottle. Makes 1 cup, which should last three months refrigerated.

Dr. Colbert's Healthy Smoothie

If you feel you are too busy to eat breakfast, here's an easy recipe for a kefir and fruit smoothie that only takes two minutes to prepare. Combine the following ingredients in a blender for a healthy snack:

- 8 oz. low-fat coconut kefir, cultured coconut milk, or low-fat coconut milk* (also for midmorning or midafternoon snack only; for evening snack, use 4 oz. water and 4 oz. coconut milk, cultured coconut milk, or coconut kefir)

- ¼ cup frozen blueberries, blackberries, strawberries, or raspberries (omit for evening snack)

- 1–2 Tbsp. ground flaxseeds (omit for evening snack)

- 1 scoop of chocolate- or vanilla-flavored egg white protein or whey protein powder or plant protein

* Make sure that the coconut milk has only 80 calories per cup.

Note: You can find more recipes like these at www.thecandodiet.com.

Coconut milk and fruit
(blend coconut milk with fruit)

- So Delicious Coconut Milk Kefir, So Delicious Cultured Coconut Milk, low-fat plain or vanilla: 8 ounces

- One medium apple

Cheese, fruit, and nuts

- 1–2 wedges of low-fat Laughing Cow cheese with 1 medium Granny Smith apple and 5–10 pecans, walnuts, almonds, or macadamia nuts

Appendix B

RESOURCE GUIDE

Most of the products mentioned throughout this book are offered through Dr. Colbert's Divine Health Wellness Center or are available at your local health food store.

Divine Health Nutritional Products
1908 Boothe Circle
Longwood, FL 32750
Phone: (407) 331-7007
Web site: www.drcolbert.com
E-mail: info@drcolbert.com

Maintenance nutritional supplements
- Divine Health Multivitamin
- Divine Health Living Multivitamin
- Divine Health Fiber Formula

Omega oils
- Divine Health Living Omega

Recommended natural sweeteners
- Chicory
- Stevia
- Just Like Sugar
- Coconut sugar
- Tagatose

Protein powders
- Divine Health Plant Protein
- Divine Health Living Protein
- Egg white protein powder

Supplements for weight loss
- Irvingia
- PGX fiber
- Living Green Tea with EGCG
- Living Green Coffee Bean
- Meratrim (Metabolic Lean)
- MBS 360: contains green coffee bean, green tea, EGCG, and Irvingia (available at www.mbs360.tv)

Supplements for thyroid support
- Metabolic Advantage
- Iodine Synergy

To curb food cravings
- Serotonin Max
- N-acetyl-tyrosine
- 5-HTP

Other supplements
- Beta TCP
- Divine Health Probiotic

- Divine Health Fiber Formula
- Vitamin D_3
- Cellgevity
- Living PQQ

OTHER RESOURCES

- ALCAT Food Sensitivity Test

- For knowledgeable doctors in bioidentical hormone replacement (make sure they are board certified in anti-aging): www .worldhealth.net

- Grissini breadsticks

- Pharmacy that carries hCG sublingual tabs (Pharmacy Specialists, (407) 260-7002

Appendix C

CONSENT FORM FOR THE RAPID WAIST CONTROL DIET

I, _____ (print name), understand that the Rapid Waist Reduction Diet has requirements, contraindications, and possible side effects. Please initial after each statement

- I understand that the FDA has *not* approved hCG for weight loss and that there is no medical data that supports the use of hCG for weight-loss purposes. ___

- I understand that I will be required to have current (within one month of beginning the RWRD program) lab test results on my chart. These tests are performed to rule out any conditions that could be worsened by the stringent caloric restriction and/or the administration of sublingual hCG in the RWRD program. ___

- I agree to report any problems or side effects that occur within the time frame of treatment to my medical professionals. ___

- I understand that I must have an established relationship with a primary care provider before starting this program. ___

- I understand that I must consult with my primary care provider to receive refills on medications that were prescribed by them. Doing so will help minimize confusion between patients and medical providers. ___

- I understand that the following conditions may prohibit intake of a low-calorie diet: ___

  - Severe liver disease (may require a low-protein diet)
  - Severe kidney disease (may require a low-protein diet)
  - Active peptic ulcer disease
  - Active cancers
  - Pregnancy, actively trying to become pregnant, or currently breast feeding
  - Eating disorder (e.g., anorexia nervosa or bulimia)
  - Severe psychiatric disturbance (e.g., major depression and/or suicide attempts, bipolar disorder, or psychosis)
  - Corticosteroid therapy greater than 20 milligrams a day

- Chronic illicit drug usage, addictions, alcoholism, substance abuse
- History of recent myocardial infarction (MI)/heart attack
- History of CVAs and/or TIAs (stroke)
- Uncontrolled seizures
- Unstable angina, clotting disorders, or DVT/PE
- Severe diabetes

- I understand that failure to comply with protocols—including keeping my primary care physician advised of my medical history, this regimen, and any changes in my condition—may predispose me to develop gallbladder disease, sabotage my weight-loss goals, or cause other harm. ___

- I understand the side effects of hCG administration and a low-calorie/nonfat diet can include dizziness, light-headedness, and lowered blood pressure. ___

- I understand that my blood pressure must be checked at least two times a week. ___

- I understand that I must be under the care of my primary care physician during the entire cycle of hCG supplementation (four to six weeks). ___

- I understand that taking diuretics, anti-inflammatory drugs, or Coumadin will require monitoring blood tests, as determined by my physician. ___

- I understand that there is a limit of 1,000 calories allowed daily on this diet. ___

- I understand that increasing my caloric intake could alter the results and increase medical risks. ___

- I understand that cheating by eating sugary or fatty foods while on phase one can be harmful and may predispose me to forming gallstones. ___

- I consent to taking sublingual hCG. I agree to be monitored by medical professionals during my weight-loss treatment period. My primary care provider will also monitor any medical condition not related to the RWRD. ___

I, _____ (print name), understand the potential risk of this program and agree to abide by the above guidelines.

Signed: _____

Date: _____

Witnessed: _____

Date: _____

Notes

Introduction—It's All About "Waist Management"

1. Centers for Disease Control and Prevention (CDC), "FastStats: Obesity and Overweight," http://www.cdc.gov/nchs/fastats/overwt.htm (accessed November 19, 2012).

1—The Obesity Epidemic

1. Wikipedia, s.v. "Super Size Me," http://en.wikipedia.org/wiki/Supersize_me (accessed November 19, 2012).

2. Mary Clare Jalonick, "Obesity Rates Still Rising," *Huffington Post*, July 7, 2011, http://www.huffingtonpost.com/2011/07/07/obesity-states-rates_n_892181.html (accessed November 1, 2011).

3. Centers for Disease Control and Prevention (CDC), "Overweight and Obesity: U.S. Obesity Trends," http://www.cdc.gov/obesity/data/trends.html (accessed November 1, 2011).

4. Ali H. Mokdad, James S. Marks, Donna F. Stroup, and Julie L. Gerberding, "Actual Causes of Death in the United States, 2000," *Journal of the American Medical Association* 291, no. 10 (March 10, 2004): 1238–1245.

5. Catherine Pearson, "Smoking Rates: Pack-A-Day Smoking Is Down Dramatically," *Huffington Post*, March 16, 2011, http://www.huffingtonpost.com/2011/03/16/smoking-rates-_n_835536.html (accessed November 19, 2012).

6. Associated Press, "Obesity Rates in U.S. Leveling Off," MSNBC.com, November 28, 2007, http://www.msnbc.msn.com/id/22007477/ns/health-diet_and_nutrition/t/obesity-rates-us-leveling (accessed November 19, 2012).

7. Centers for Disease Control and Prevention (CDC), "Overweight and Obesity: Defining Overweight and Obesity," http://www.cdc.gov/obesity/defining.html (accessed November 19, 2012).

8. Osama Hamdy, "Obesity," Medscape.com, September 24, 2012, http://emedicine.medscape.com/article/123702-overview (accessed November 19, 2012).

9. E. A. Finkelstein, J. G. Trogdon, J. W. Cohen, and W. Dietz, "Annual Medical Spending Attributable to Obesity: Payer- and Science-Specific Estimates," *Health Affairs* 28, no. 5 (2009): w822–w831, as referenced in Weight-Control Information Network, National Institute of Diabetes and

Digestive and Kidney Diseases (NIDDK), "Overweight and Obesity Statistics: Economic Costs Related to Overweight and Obesity," http://win .niddk.nih.gov/statistics/#what (accessed November 1, 2011).

10. ScienceDaily.com, "Breast Cancer More Aggressive in Obese Women, Study Suggests," March 14, 2008, http://www.sciencedaily.com/ releases/2008/03/080314085045.htm (accessed November 19, 2012).

11. Jillita Horton, "Why Obesity Increases Risk of Uterine Cancer," August 26, 2010, http://voices.yahoo.com/why-obesity-increases-risk -uterine-cancer-6650104.html (accessed November 19, 2012).

12. CBSNews.com, "Birth Defects Linked to Obesity," April 6, 2010, http://www.cbsnews.com/2100-204_162-548286.html (accessed November 19, 2012).

13. Eric Schlosser, *Fast Food Nation* (New York: Houghton Mifflin, 2001), 3, 242.

14. Woodruff Health Sciences Center, "Excess Fat Puts Patients with Type 2 Diabetes at Greater Risk," March 26, 2009, http://shared.web .emory.edu/whsc/news/releases/2009/03/excess-fat-puts-diabetic-patients -at-risk.html (accessed November 1, 2011).

15. ScienceDaily.com, "Obesity Increases Cancer Risk, Analysis of Hundreds of Studies Shows," February 17, 2008, http://www.sciencedaily .com/releases/2008/02/080217211802.htm (accessed November 19, 2012).

16. The Healthier Life.com, "GERD: Obesity Can Increase Your Risk of Acid Reflux Disease," March 29, 2006, http://www.thehealthierlife .co.uk/natural-health-articles/digestive-problems/gerd-obesity-increase -risk-00212.html (accessed November 19, 2012).

17. Frank Mangano, "The Obesity-Hypertension Connection: Your Weight May Be Putting You at Risk," NaturalNews.com, July 27, 2009, http://www.naturalnews.com/026702_weight_blood_pressure.html (accessed November 19, 2012).

18. A. J. Stunkard, T. I. Sorensen, C. Hanis, et al., "An Adoption Study of Human Obesity," *New England Journal of Medicine* 314, no. 4 (January 23, 1986): 193–198.

19. National Heart, Lung, and Blood Institute, National Institutes of Health, "What Causes Overweight and Obesity?", http://www.nhlbi.nih .gov/health/health-topics/topics/obe/causes.html (accessed November 19, 2012).

20. Pamela Peeke, *Fight Fat After Forty* (New York: Viking, 2000), 58.

2—Culprit #1: Inflammation

1. Wikipedia.org, s.v. "List of Wildfires: North America," http://en.wikipedia.org/wiki/List_of_wildfires#North_America (accessed November 19, 2012).

2. H. Du, D. L. van der A, M. M. van Bakel, et al., "Glycemic Index and Glycemic Load in Relation to Food and Nutrient Intake and Metabolic Risk Factors in a Dutch Population," *American Journal of Clinical Nutrition* 87, no. 3 (March 2008): 655–661.

3. G. Davi, M. T. Guagnano, G. Ciabattoni, et al., "Platelet Activation in Obese Women: Role of Inflammation and Oxidant Stress," *Journal of the American Medical Association* 288, no. 16 (October 23–30, 2002): 2008–2014.

4. B. B. Duncan, M. I. Schmidt, L. E. Chambless, A. R. Folsom, and G. Heiss, "Atherosclerosis Risk in Communities Study Investigators: Inflammation Markers Predict Increased Weight Gain in Smoking Quitters," *Obesity Research* 11, no. 11 (November 2003): 1339–1344; and E. Barinas-Mitchell, M. Cushman, E. N. Meilahn, R. P. Tracy, and L. H. Kuller, "Serum Levels of C-Reactive Protein Are Associated With Obesity, Weight Gain, and Hormone Replacement Therapy in Healthy Postmenopausal Women," *American Journal of Epidemiology* 153, no. 11 (June 2001): 1094–1101.

5. G. Engstrom, B. Hedblad, L. Stavenow, P. Lind, L. Janzon, and F. Lindgarde, "Inflammation-Sensitive Plasma Proteins Are Associated With Future Weight Gain," *Diabetes* 52, no. 8 (August 2003): 2097–2101.

6. Clara Felix, *All About Omega-3 Oils* (Garden City, NY: Avery Publishing, 1998), 32.

7. Jeanie Lerche Davis, "Top 10 Foods With Trans Fats," WebMD.com, May 21, 2004, http://www.webmd.com/diet/features/top-10-foods-with-trans-fats (accessed November 19, 2012).

8. William Davis, *Wheat Belly* (New York: Rodale, 2011), 14.

9. H. C. Broeck, H. C. de Jong, E. M. Salentijn, et al., "Presence of Celiac Disease Epitopes in Modern and Old Hexaploid Wheat Varieties: Wheat Breeding May Have Contributed to Increased Prevalence of Celiac Disease," *Theoretical and Applied Genetics* 121, no. 8 (November 2010): 1527–1539, as referenced in Davis, *Wheat Belly*, 26.

10. Davis, *Wheat Belly*, 35.

11. Ibid., 36, 53–54.

12. Ibid., 45.

13. Marian Burros, "Stores Say Wild Salmon, but Tests Say Farm Bred," *New York Times*, April 10, 2005, http://www.nytimes

.com/2005/04/10/dining/10salmon.html?scp=1&sq=stores+say+
wild+salmon&st=nyt&_r=0 (accessed November 19, 2012).

3—Culprit #2: Carbs—Especially Wheat

1. Davis, *Wheat Belly*, 56.

2. Ibid., 103.

3. Ibid., 70.

4. US Department of Health and Human Services, *Dietary Guidelines for Americans, 2005*, 6th ed. (Washington DC: U.S. Government Printing Office, 2005).

5. Neal Bernard, *Breaking the Food Seduction* (New York: St. Martin's Press, 2003), 32.

6. Davis, *Wheat Belly*, 32–33.

7. John Casey, "The Hidden Ingredient That Can Sabotage Your Diet," MedicineNet.com, http://www.medicinenet.com/script/main/art.asp?articlekey=56589 (accessed November 20, 2012).

8. Becky Hand, "The Hunt for Hidden Sugar," BabyFit.com, http://babyfit.sparkpeople.com/articles.asp?id=685 (accessed November 20, 2012).

9. MyFoxNY.com, "Teens' Sugar Intake Poses Health Risks," January 12, 2011, http://www.myfoxny.com/story/17425214/teens-sugar-intake-raises-health-risks (accessed November 20, 2012).

10. Centers for Disease Control and Prevention, "Overweight and Obesity: Adult Obesity Facts," http://www.cdc.gov/obesity/data/adult.html (accessed January 14, 2013); Centers for Disease Control and Prevention, "National Diabetes Month—November 2012," *Morbidity and Mortality Weekly Report* 61, no. 43 (November 2, 2012): 869, http://www.cdc.gov/mmwr/preview/mmwrhtml/mm6143a1.htm (accessed January 14, 2013).

11. Sucralose.org, "Your Questions Answered," http://www.sucralose.org/questions/ (accessed November 20, 2012).

12. Sally Fallon Morell and Rami Nagel, "Agave Nectar: Worse Than We Thought," *Wise Traditions*, Spring 2009, 44–51, http://www.westonaprice.org/modern-foods/agave-nectar-worse-than-we-thought (accessed November 20, 2012).

13. Drugs.com, "Spherix Announces Statistically Significant Results in Phase 3 Study With D-tagatose in Type 2 Diabetics," October 2010, http://www.drugs.com/clinical_trials/spherix-announces-statistically-significant-results-phase-3-study-d-tagatose-type-2-diabetes-10296.html (accessed January 14, 2013).

4—Your Waistline Is Your Lifeline

1. Linda K. "Tallest, Fastest, Longest: Top 10 Roller Coasters in America," *Uptake* (blog), April 29, 2009, http://attractions.uptake.com/blog/top-10-roller-coasters-4014.html (accessed November 20, 2012).

2. Lauren Muney, "Top 10 Excuses for Falling Off the Diet/Fitness Wagon—and Answers for Them," PhysicalMind.com, http://www.physicalmind.com/articles.html (accessed November 20, 2012).

3. Centers for Disease Control and Prevention (CDC), "Overweight and Obesity: Defining Overweight and Obesity."

4. Youfa Wang, Eric B. Rimm, Meir J. Stampfer, Walter C. Willett, and Frank B. Hu, "Comparison of Abdominal Adiposty and Overall Obesity in Predicting Risk of Type 2 Diabetes Among Men," *American Journal of Clinical Nutrition* 81, No. 3 (2005): 555–563.

5—Forget the Number on the Scale

1. Amanda Spake, "The Belly Burden," *U.S. News & World Report*, November 20, 2005, http://health.usnews.com/usnews/health/articles/051128/28waist.htm (accessed November 20, 2012).

2. Krisha McCoy, "Your Body Fat Percentage: What Does It Mean?", BeliefNet.com, July 2008, http://www.beliefnet.com/healthandhealing/getcontent.aspx?cid=41373 (accessed November 20, 2012).

8—Rapid Waist Reduction Diet, Phase Two

1. American College of Obstetricians and Gynecologists, "Nutrition During Pregnancy," patient education information sheet, June 2008.

2. L. R. Goldman, M. W. Shannon, and American Academy of Pediatrics: Committee on Environmental Health, "Technical Report: Mercury in the Environment: Implications for Pediatricians," *Pediatrics* 108, no. 1 (July 2001): 197–205.

9—Treats and Cheats

1. Jennie Brand-Miller, Thomas M. S. Wolever, Kay Foster-Powell, and Stephen Colagiuri, *The New Glucose Revolution*, 3rd ed. (New York: Marlow & Co., 2007), 86.

2. Charles Stuart Platkin, *The Automatic Diet* (New York: Hudson Street Press, 2005), 92.

3. M. Conceicao de Oliveira, R. Sichieri, and A. Sanchez, "Weight Loss Association With a Daily Intake of Three Apples or Three Pears Among Overweight Women," *Nutrition* 19, no. 3 (2003): 253–256.

4. Judith J. Wurtman and Nina Frusztajer Marquis, *The Serotonin Power Diet* (New York: Rodale, 2006), 15.

5. Ibid., 66–68.

10—EATING OUT AND GROCERY SHOPPING

1. National Restaurant Association, "Restaurant Industry Sales Turn Positive in 2011 After Three Tough Years," PRNewswire, February 1, 2011, http://multivu.prnewswire.com/mnr/national-restaurant -association/42965/ (accessed November 26, 2012).

2. National Restaurant Association, "National Restaurant Association's First-of-Its-Kind 'Kids LiveWell' Initiative Showcases Restaurants' Healthful Menu Options for Children," press release, July 13, 2011, http://www.restaurant.org/pressroom/pressrelease/?ID=2136 (accessed November 26, 2012).

3. Rich Pirog, Timothy Van Pelt, Kamyar Enshayan, and Ellen Cook, "Food, Fuel, and Freeways: An Iowa Perspective on How Far Food Travels, Fuel Usage, and Greenhouse Gas Emissions," Leopold Center for Sustainable Agriculture, June 2001, http://www.leopold.iastate.edu/pubs -and-papers/2001-06-food-fuel-freeways (accessed November 9, 2011).

4. SupermarketGuru.com, "The Things You Need to Know About Frozen Dinners," April 4, 2007, http://archive.supermarketguru.com/ page.cfm/32858 (accessed November 26, 2012).

11—SUPPLEMENTS THAT SUPPORT WEIGHT LOSS AND BURN BELLY FAT

1. Michael Johnsen, "Obesity Epidemic Feeds Weight-Loss Product Sales," DrugStoreNews.com, January 5, 2011, http://www.drugstorenews .com/article/obesity-epidemic-feeds-weight-loss-product-sales (accessed November 26, 2012).

2. Stephen Bent, Thomas N. Tiedt, Michelle C. Odden, and Michael G. Shlipak, "The Relative Safety of Ephedra Compared With Other Herbal Products," *Annals of Internal Medicine* 138, no. 6 (March 18, 2003): 468–471, http://annals.org/article.aspx?articleid=716166 (accessed November 26, 2012).

3. Associated Press, "FDA Warns Consumers to Avoid Brazilian Diet Pills," USAToday.com, January 13, 2006, http://usatoday30.usatoday.com/ news/health/2006-01-13-brazilian-diet-pills_x.htm (accessed November 26, 2012).

4. Ano Lobb, "Hepatoxicity Associated With Weight-Loss Supplements: A Case for Better Post-Marketing Surveillance, *World Journal of*

Gastroenterology 15, no. 14 (April 14, 2009): 1786–1787, http://www.ncbi
.nlm.nih.gov/pmc/articles/PMC2668789/ (accessed November 26, 2012).

5. Julius Goepp, "Critical Need for a Multi-Modal Approach to
Combat Obesity," *Life Extension*, June 2009, http://www.lef.org/
magazine/mag2009/jun2009_Multi-Modal-Approach-To-Combat
-Obesity_01.htm (accessed November 26, 2012).

6. P. Chantre and D. Lairon, "Recent Findings of Green Tea Extract
AR25 (Exolise) and Its Activity for the Treatment of Obesity," *Phytomed-
icine* 9, no. 1 (2002): 3–8.

7. Goepp, "Critical Need for a Multi-Modal Approach to Combat
Obesity."

8. LifeExtension.org, "Journal Abstracts: Green Coffee Bean Extract,"
Life Extension Magazine, February 2012, http://www.lef.org/magazine/
mag2012/abstracts/feb2012_Green-Coffee-Bean-Extract_04.htm
(accessed November 26, 2012).

9. Douglas Laboratories, "Metabolic Lean: Weight Management Formula," product data sheet, June 2012, http://www.douglaslabs.com/pdf/
pds/201350.pdf (accessed January 15, 2013).

10. American Thyroid Association, "Iodine Deficiency," http://www
.thyroid.org/iodine-deficiency/ (accessed November 26, 2012).

11. Lisa Bolton, Americus Reed II, Kevin G. Volpp, and Katrina Arm-
strong, "How Does Drug and Supplement Marketing Affect a Healthy
Lifestyle?" *Journal of Consumer Research* 34 (February 2008).

12. J. A. Marlett, M. I. McBurney, J. L. Slavin, and American Dietetic
Association, "Position of the American Dietetic Association: Health
Implications of Dietary Fiber," *Journal of the American Dietetic Associa-
tion* 102, no. 7 (2002): 993–1000.

13. N. C. Howarth, E. Saltzman, and S. B. Roberts, "Dietary Fiber and
Weight Regulation," *Nutrition Review* 59, no. 5 (2001): 129–138.

14. Life Extension, "Obesity: Strategies to Fight a Rising Epidemic,"
http://www.lef.org/protocols/metabolic_health/obesity_01.htm (accessed
November 26, 2012).

15. Judith N. Ngondi, Blanche C. Etoundi, Christine B. Nyangono,
Carl M. F. Mbofung, and Julius E. Oben, "IGOB131, a Novel Seed Extract
of the West African Plant Irvingia Gabonensis, Significantly Reduces
Body Weight and Improves Metabolic Parameters in Overweight
Humans in a Randomized Double-Blind Placebo Controlled Investigation," *Lipids in Health and Disease* 8, no. 7 (March 2009): http://www
.lipidworld.com/content/8/1/7 (accessed November 26, 2012).

16. Hoodia Advice, "The Science of Hoodia," http://www.hoodia
-advice.org/hoodia-plant.html (accessed November 26, 2012).

17. Tom Mangold, "Sampling the Kalahari Hoodia Diet," BBC News, May 30, 2003, http://news.bbc.co.uk/2/hi/programmes/correspondent/2947810.stm (accessed November 26, 2012).

12—THE IMPORTANCE OF ACTIVITY

1. TMZ.com, "Janet in Shape and in 'Control,'" July 27, 2006, http://www.tmz.com/2006/07/17/janet-in-shape-and-in-control/ (accessed November 26, 2012).

2. Rob Carnevale, "Bruce Willis: Die Hard 4.0," BBC, July 2, 2007, http://www.bbc.co.uk/films/2007/07/02/bruce_willis_die_hard_4_2007_interview.shtml (accessed November 26, 2012).

3. Starpulse.com, "Memorable Celebrity Quotes," January 16, 2008, http://www.starpulse.com/news/index.php/2008/01/16/memorable_celebrity_quotes_118 (accessed November 26, 2012).

4. Mirelle Agaman, "Exclusive: Serena Williams Talks to Star!," *Star*, May 4, 2007, http://www.starmagazine.com/news/exclusive-serena-williams-talks-star (accessed November 9, 2011).

5. Stephen Miller, "Jack LaLanne, Media Fitness Guru, Dies at 96," *Wall Street Journal*, January 24, 2011, http://online.wsj.com/article/SB10001424052748703398504576100923135057068.html (accessed November 26, 2012).

6. Centers for Disease Control and Prevention (CDC), "U.S. Physical Activity Statistics," http://apps.nccd.cdc.gov/PASurveillance/StateSumV.asp (accessed November 26, 2012).

7. Jacqueline Stenson, "Excuses, Excuses," MSNBC.com, December 16, 2004, http://www.msnbc.msn.com/id/6391079/ns/health-fitness/t/excuses-excuses/ (accessed November 26, 2012); Chad Clark, "Functional Exercise: Top 10 List of Reasons Why People Don't Exercise," http://pt-connections.com/topfit/publish/printer_functional_exercise_top_10_reasons.shtml (accessed November 9, 2011).

8. Centers for Disease Control and Prevention (CDC), "Physical Activity for Everyone," http://www.cdc.gov/physicalactivity/everyone/guidelines/adults.html (accessed November 26, 2012).

9. Jennifer Corbett Dooren, "New Exercise Goal: 60 Minutes a Day," *Wall Street Journal*, March 24, 2010, http://online.wsj.com/article/SB10001424052748704896104575140011148266470.html (accessed November 26, 2012).

10. David Zinczenko with Matt Goulding, *Eat This, Not That!* (New York: Rodale Books, 2008), 113.

11. Associated Baptist Press, "70-Year-Old Swims English Channel to Promote Church's Ministry in Haiti," September 1, 2004, http://www

.abpnews.com/archives/item/1863-70-year-old-swims-english-channel-to
-promote-churchs-ministry-in-haiti (accessed November 27, 2012).

12. J. A. Levine, L. M. Lanningham-Foster, S. K. McCrady, et al.,
"Interindividual Variation in Posture Allocation: Possible Role in Human
Obesity," *Science* 307, no. 5709 (January 28, 2005): 584–586.

13. Centers for Disease Control and Prevention, "How Much Physical
Activity Do Adults Need?", December 1, 2011, http://www.cdc.gov/
physicalactivity/everyone/guidelines/adults.html (accessed November 27,
2012).

14. C. A. Slentz, B. D. Duscha, J. L. Johnson, et al., "Effects of the
Amount of Exercise on Body Weight, Body Composition, and Measures
of Central Obesity," *Archives of Internal Medicine* 164, no. 1 (January 12,
2004): 31–39.

15. Caroline J. Cedarquist, "Fitness With Fido: A Healthy Pastime for
Dog Owners," NewsBlaze.com, January 10, 2006, http://newsblaze.com/
story/20060110091932nnnn.nb/topstory.html (accessed November 27,
2012).

16. Berit L. Heitmann and Peder Frederiksen, "Thigh Circumference
and Risk of Heart Disease and Premature Death: Prospective Cohort
Study," *British Medical Journal* 339 (September 3, 2009):http://www.bmj
.com/content/339/bmj.b3292 (accessed November 27, 2012).

17. Peter Jaret, "A Healthy Mix of Rest and Motion," *New York Times*,
May 3, 2007, http://tinyurl.com/c7zxot3 (accessed November 27, 2012).

18. K. N. Boutelle and D. S. Kirschenbaum, "Further Support for Consistent Self-Monitoring as a Vital Component of Successful Weight Control," *Obesity Research* 6, no. 3 (May 1998): 219–224, http://www.ncbi
.nlm.nih.gov/pubmed/9618126 (accessed November 27, 2012).

Index

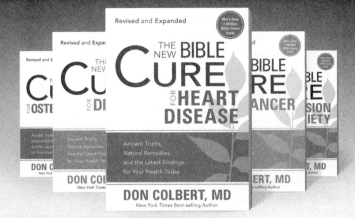

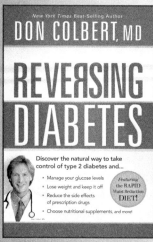
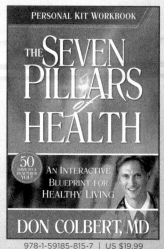